HAD ELLIS ISLAND WASHED AWAY

*A history of Ellis Island and
why it still matters today*

Brett Moyer

Copyright © 2022 Brett Moyer

All rights reserved

The characters and events portrayed in this book are fictitious. Any similarity to real persons, living or dead, is coincidental and not intended by the author.

No part of this book may be reproduced, or stored in a retrieval system, or transmitted in any form or by any means, electronic, mechanical, photocopying, recording, or otherwise, without express written permission of the publisher.

ISBN-13: 9798430921378

Printed in the United States of America

*To my first history teachers, Meda and Todd Moyer
& Bill Yost.*

*Also by Brett Moyer
Had Lincoln Lived*

CONTENTS

Title Page	1
Copyright	2
Dedication	3
Introduction	7
Part I: Native Americans to the New Americans: Pre-Ellis Island	13
Chapter 1: Oyster Island	14
Chapter 2: Farm to Famine	23
Chapter 3: Entering the Castle	31
Part II: The Beginnings of Ellis Island	47
Chapter 4: Oyster Island to Ellis Island	48
Chapter 5: Able Bodied Workers	61
Chapter 6: The Y in the Road	79
Part III: The End of an Era of Ellis Island Immigration	103
Chapter 7: The End of Ellis Immigration	104
Chapter 8: Island of Hope - Forgotten	113

Chapter 9: Why it Matters Today	119
Afterword	129
Acknowledgement	133
Bibliography	135
About The Author	139

INTRODUCTION

On a chilly spring morning, as the thick fog clears over the sparkling Hudson River, an island set in history appears. It has modern day skyscrapers bowing to it in the middle of the harbor.

I am making my way across the quarter mile steel-grated bridge connecting Liberty State Park, New Jersey to Ellis Island – a bridge many people are puzzled and surprised even exists to service the Island today.

I realize there is a story that is much larger than I can ever begin to tell about the Island I am journeying towards. This is the story of how one island changed the lives of millions of people: from the immigrants who spent anxious hours on the Island hoping to live the American dream to those doctors and immigration personnel who had dedicated themselves to make the system work.

I have the wonderful privilege of walking this bridge as a docent with Save Ellis Island, a non-profit park partner of the National Parks Service that is dedicated to the restoration of the south side of the Island. I have gotten to enjoy seeing the peaceful pre-dawn reds over the city turn to pinks as visitors, who wish to walk in the footsteps of their ancestors, begin to make their way to the Island. My role has allowed me to give medical history tours for the last six years to thousands of tourists in the abandoned immigrant hospitals on the south side of the Island. I have made it a goal to end each of my tours by telling my guests that if they take anything from it, they should not take my bad jokes but perhaps take the humility of said space.

The idea of Ellis Island being one of the most famous ports of entry in the world slipping below the tides of the Hudson River may seem preposterous. However, this is more of a story of what could have been had Ellis Island never opened to allow in those immigrants seeking a better life. What if the beautiful Island that welcomed over sixteen million immigrants, and today receives over two million visitors a year, never grew from its humble beginnings from three acres just above the wavy tide to a sprawling twenty-seven-and-a-half-acre National Park?

As Emma Lazarus would state in her famous poem, "give me your tired, your poor, your huddled masses yearning to breathe free, the wretched refuse of your teeming shore, send these, the homeless, tempest-tossed, to me: I lift my lamp beside the golden door."[1] This inscription, which is beset on the Statue of Liberty today, shows the drive and sacrifice of these 'huddled masses' of immigrants who took a shot at the American dream in this new world.

Ever since the departure from the pristine and majestic Garden of Eden, humans have been on the move. The quest has been driven by the search for plentiful resources, freedom, and safety. America would grow from small pockets of settlements of Native Americans to small port cities and then to thirteen colonies bordering the Atlantic Ocean. This expansion would set up America to be the land of opportunity, offering hope to those immigrants yearning to breathe free.

Today, whether one travels from Battery Park at the tip of Manhattan, New York, or from Liberty State Park by the shores of New Jersey, one cannot help but almost overlook Ellis Island dwarfed next to Lady Liberty on Bedloe's Island. While these two islands are separated by a mere .6 nautical miles, many visitors of Lady Liberty would not even brave the often-choppy waters to get off the ferryboat to visit the historic immigration museum – such a sharp contrast from how things were almost a hundred years ago. Before, immigrants would bet their whole lives to travel thousands of nautical miles just to kiss the ground of Ellis Island.

For many of the early immigrants, their journey across the Atlantic could take a few months on sail powered-ships and their destination was not always certain. However, by the time of Ellis Island opening in 1892, the trip across would be cut to a short week at top speed using state of the art steam powered-ships.[2] The trips could be extended though as these large steam ships would make many stops before they finally embarked on the journey across the Atlantic. As a consequence, many of the passengers would be in steerage for weeks in huddled masses dreaming of their final destination.

As a vessel would turn into the mouth of the Hudson, and the first lights of shore lay out, travelling immigrants would be filled with equal parts joy and anxiety, including thoughts of all that might be in store for them. This notwithstanding, they would fight for a view of their new home, hungry for new opportunities, and what would be next in their stories.

Although the prized statistics say that one in three Americans can trace their ancestry to Ellis Island, with the passing of each and every year, the history of Ellis Island becomes more and more a waning distant remembrance. People's memories of their ancestors betting it all on this dream begins to fade in old scrapbooks and family trees long since forgotten and splintered. The statistics also weaken as we step further away in time from the closing of the Island during a cold November winter afternoon of 1954 when the last detainee would be released.

This closing year would also be decades removed from the peak years of immigration on the Island.

So had this Island never been raised, it would have been a different landscape not only for the New York skyline but also the world. Let me illustrate how would your voyage look.

On a cool autumn morning, if you would have the chance to board one of the ferryboats in the Hudson River, the packed vessel would be quite hushed as you made your way across the river. It would be smooth sailing as no need for countless other vessels to support the rush of daily commuters resulting in no foamy wake for your trip.

The skyline ahead would perhaps never have stretched beyond the lower tip of Manhattan and green sheep pastures would still stream up the hilly island as far as the eye can see. And if the Statue of Liberty would still have ever been raised to welcome people to this quiet city, you may notice a small island a short distance north of her in the Hudson. This island would only be noticeable at a distance during calm tides. This pile of sharp rocks would have only ever been famous for the hangings of pirates conducted there and not as the island that would mark the entry for millions.

Without Ellis Island, the millions of immigrants who would have streamed into New

York certainly had other options to gain entry to these 'streets of gold' in America. However, the question is: would they have even made the risk?

Without this Island, this place, the country we know today would have been very different. These streets would have been plagued with their fellow countrymen sick and ill, less prepared for the real 'Island of Tears' and a nation that would look very different from the America we know today. How fortunate we are that as we cross the Hudson River today, we have tunnels, bridges, and ferry's galore – all built by these millions who streamed to this land of opportunity. How fortunate that the island of rocks did not slip below the waters of the Hudson.

PART I: NATIVE AMERICANS TO THE NEW AMERICANS: PRE-ELLIS ISLAND

CHAPTER 1: OYSTER ISLAND

> "We become not a melting pot but a beautiful mosaic. Different people, different beliefs, different yearnings, different hopes, different dreams."
>
> – Jimmy Carter

As the large English-built SS Nevada slowly drifted into the New York Harbor at the end of 1891, it was about to make history. The early steam vessel built by "Palmer's Shipbuilding & Iron Co. in 1868" had made the trip across the icy cold Atlantic, carrying many Irish Immigrants looking to build a new life in America.[3] The most famous on board, with arrival slated for New Year's Day of 1892, would not be that of a world-famous scientist, wealthy industrialist, or a king; it would be that of a humble freckled thirteen-year-old, Annie Moore. Her story would only be the beginning of what would be Ellis Island. To fully understand how pivotal and important this moment was to the future of immigration, we need to look back how it all began at Ellis Island, the Island of Hope.

As far back as the ice age, the earliest known settlers of this region would be the Algonquian tribes. These early tribes would be spread out throughout the whole of New England. But in its lower portion, one of the most famous tribes in the New York Harbors using these islands for fishing would be that of the Lenape. The original New Yorkers in the region "known as the Lenape, were, at first, mostly amicable and welcoming, according to historical records. They shared the land and were known for their trade of guns, beads and wool for beaver furs." [4] As the story goes, the Dutch were even able to strike one of the greatest real-estate deals in New York history with this group. The Dutch colonists were able to purchase Manhattan Island from the Lenape in 1626 for a whole $24 in trade. According to Bloomberg, the land value of Manhattan tops the scales at $1.74 trillion today.

However, in the early period of American history, the Lenape men would be often found in their small boats bobbing in the Hudson River. Here, they would be found laying hand-woven nets on the rivers for fishing and harvesting the abundant supply of fish and oysters in the region to sustain themselves. The shells of the oysters would even be able to serve as an early currency in the region. This supply of protein rich food and plentiful resources made the region more attractive to new settlers looking to survive in this new land.

From its early days and abundant supply of oyster, the Ellis Island we know today would receive its first name from the Dutch: Oyster Island.

Who would have thought that the oyster would have been the most famous food in New York, long before the "quintessential New York City food, pizza, hot pretzels, bagels, and hot dogs?"[5] These early oysters were not only in great quantity but also much larger in size – a thought that would make any chef giddy today. As the New York Harbor was dotted with numerous small islands, these brackish waters would prove to be a great ecosystem for the oysters to grow. The nearly twenty-eight acre island we know today would grow from these humble roots.

With its fertile soils and shallow clean waters, the New York region would prove to be an excellent environment for all to make a living and prosper. The Lenape also understood the ecology of this wonderful supply – returning the used shells back to the waters to help spawn the next generation of oysters to support those that would follow.

As fishermen would begin to make the New York harbor their treasure trove, they would have to work quickly to harvest their crop in between a growing ferry service traversing the harbor. The demand was not only from the growing American colonies, but also for the increasing European populations.

As time would pass, the population of oysters would significantly drop from earlier days because of commercialization of fishing over the decades and the pollution of the rivers. By the 20th century, oysters harvested in this region would be considered too polluted to even be eaten. It was not until the early 1970's and the passage of the Clean Water Act of 1972 that efforts to save this valuable part of the river were implemented. Today, efforts remain underway to help restore this amazing creature to the harbor as a single oyster is able to filter and clean up to fifty gallons of water a day – an ever-important need for the Hudson River and surrounding ecosystems.

But the Island, and not the humble oyster which made the region famous, is the real purpose of our tale. So where does the name Ellis finally come in if this Island had always been called the Oyster Island?

Through the purchase of Manhattan by the Dutch, the man who we associate with the Island today, Samuel Ellis, would take ownership of the then three-acre island. "Samuel Ellis, who called it Oyster Island like the Dutch settlers before him, was a tavern owner and merchant who bought the island in the 1770s."[6] Samuel, of 1 Greenwich Street in lower Manhattan, would begin operations of his busy tavern on the Island on November of 1774 until his passing twenty years later.

The Island under Samuel's ownership would also be known by its other historical names such as Gulls Island and Gibbet Island. Gibbet Island, when translated in Dutch, would mean the infamous 'Gallows' that stood on the Island.

During the time of Samuel's ownership of the Island, the small rocky land mass would be used for hangings aside from inebriation at the tavern for weary sailors. "For most of the early 19th century, the [Island] was used to hang convicted pirates, criminals and mutinous sailors, and New Yorkers eventually took to calling it 'Gibbet Island' after the wooden post, or gibbet, where the bodies of the deceased were displayed."[7] The unpleasant display was a sign to any pirate or sinister criminal entering the harbor that any villainous activity would be met with a swift and unpleasant end. Ellis Island would see its last execution there in June of 1839 when "pirate and murderer Cornelius Wilhelms was hanged on the island"[8] as penalty for his crime.

Decades before the death of this pirate, as Samuel breathed his last breath, the fate of Ellis Island would be in the hands of his young daughter, Catherine Westervelt, and her unborn son to whom the Island was supposed to be passed on to. Passing the Island to Samuel's grandson was done to keep the Ellis name going, but also because women were not allowed to control property in New York until 1848.

Unfortunately, the newly-born Samuel Ellis would pass in infancy. The young daughter of Samuel would maintain ownership but not control of the Island as New York City would deed Ellis Island to New York State for militarily strategic purposes for the U.S. War Department. It would take until 1808 for New York State to pay the Ellis family $10,000 for this small island and begin building a series of fortifications in the harbor for the federal government.

From a tavern to a tower, Ellis Island would be part of a series of three strategic islands to defend the harbor. Ellis Island would be joined by Governor's Island to the east and Bedloe's Island just to the south to secure and defend the harbor from potential invasion. Given the challenges of defending the growing island of Manhattan, but also the sheer width of the Hudson, the government knew they needed a series of forts to secure this valuable island and its commerce. Nearly a third of the federal government's revenue came from the New York ports and taxes collected therefrom.

On Governor's Island stood an army fort, Fort Jay, which would be renamed Fort Columbus during the next century. This island stood as a key to defending the East River and the growing city of

Brooklyn to the far east. With eight-foot-thick stone walls and eighty powerful guns, it was considered a last line of defense should forts out near the narrows fail.

On Bedloe's Island, a star-shaped Fort Wood would be constructed as its defense. The fort would house twenty-four guns and a garrison to quickly fire on any enemy ship. The very same fort stands as part of the foundation for the Statue of Liberty today. This southern portion of the defense would stand in line with Ellis Island and her fort to be constructed.

On Ellis Island, Fort Gibson would be the defense built to secure the harbor. The early "crescent-shaped structure of wood and sod built in 1794 on the edge of what was then the island's shoreline" would be redesigned as America was on the verge of the War of 1812.[9] The newly constructed fort at Ellis Island would have over one dozen cannon at the ready and a garrison of over 180 trained men to serve its duty. The United States government had seen such a dreadful defeat at New York during the Revolutionary War that it did not want to repeat.

With hundreds of cannons and thousands of men guarding the city, the only fighting in New York State during the war would come far upstate. The closest call would be on August 18, 1814, when a small group of British warships would be seen south of the city – never adventuring closer to the see the wrath of the guns.

Between the end of the War of 1812 and the opening story of immigration at Ellis Island in 1892, the Island was used by the United States Navy for storage of large powder magazines for the ever-growing navy presence in the region. This storage would be a concern to the growing populations in New York City and Jersey City in case of deadly explosion of the unstable powder.

One such example of this danger would come in later years at a smaller island just to the west of Ellis Island, Black Tom's Island. This island would be used for powder storage in the early days of World War I on the New Jersey shores. It was "still dark in Manhattan on a Sunday morning, July 30, 1916, when the sky suddenly exploded with an unnatural brilliance" according to FBI reports.[10] German agents had been able to quickly sneak into the rail depot at Black Tom's Island and light off over an astounding two million pounds of explosives stored there. In all, three men and an infant were killed, and even the Statue of Liberty would nearly see her arm dislocated from the blast. The blast would rock the country in more ways than one, and windows would be shattered all throughout the city as the window for the United States to enter World War I was opening.

The threat of using these islands for such

military purposes clearly concerned the burgeoning populations growing nearby. However, the islands being used for such purposes were transitioning. One such island would be chosen to change from defending against intruders to welcoming immigrants. Such is the tale of Ellis Island.

CHAPTER 2: FARM TO FAMINE

> "Whether our ancestors came here on the Mayflower, on slave ships, whether they came to Ellis Island or LAX in Los Angeles, whether they came yesterday or walked this land a thousand years ago our great challenge for the 21st century is to find a way to be One America. We can meet all the other challenges if we can go forward as One America."
>
> – William J. Clinton

The story of immigration to America stretches millennia as seen in how the Native Americans were spread out across the United States and North America. Their story defines how this land was truly made to be explored. The first voyages across the seas from the days of Christopher Columbus were simply the beginning of what would become an immigration boom to discover this new uncharted territory.

So was it the knowledge of the open fertile land, the sense of freedom from persecution, riches, or just the ability to travel and adventure across the open seas that drove people to this new place? There were truly so many reasons that pushed this migration and journey into the unknown.

From the early expeditions to the new world we realize, the quest was not only in seeking discovery but in finding ways to trade easier and quicker. Large government-funded sailing expeditions would see sailors traversing these uncharted areas.

Through rolling blue seas, adventurous sailors would set out for destinations far and wide. However, they would bring with them disease and threats to the cultures they would meet. The knowledge of potential death by an unseen and often unknown disease would make those they would encounter often apprehensive to extending a warm welcome.

The understanding of the threats of deadly diseases and limited resources would often find the early Native Americans at odds with the new settlers. For those onboard the vessels bobbing towards shore, they had been warned of hostile natives. We know it was often through force, but also through shrewd negotiations and a willingness to bargain for their safety, that America would begin its growth on the eastern shores. As this new land offered respite for weary adventurers, settlements would grow and large port cities would emerge as entry points.

On the eve of the birth of America in 1775, the United States had a population of just over 2.4 million residents, nearly a quarter of which were enslaved. However, it is remarkable to note that the majority of those residents would not be crowded into the port cities in which they had immigrated originally. The largest cities of "Philadelphia [with] 38,000 [residents]; New York City, 25,000; Boston, 16,000; Charleston, 12,000; and Newport, 11,000" would make them the large urban centers and simply ports of entry.[11]

Why would early America only see five percent of its population in these port cities in 1775? If we fast forward to today, just 250 years later, over eighty percent of the United States population live in and near urban centers.[12] The statistics would also be true around the globe. In countries like England, Germany, and France, rural living was also the common way of life. So what drove this massive shift from rural to urban living over the decades?

The US Census Bureau paints a very interesting picture to help understand this overall trend over the years. "Urbanization in the United States began to increase rapidly through the 19th century, reaching 40 percent by 1900. By 1950 this reached 64%, and nearly 80% by 2000."[13] Similar statistics are true around the globe today.

To explain the trend, we need to understand first how cities were like in the past. Accounts tell of how cities were scary as people were crowded together. Countless histories detail how outbreaks would quickly decimate these early port cities in America, leaving people fleeing for the countryside. With limited medical understanding, people thought that the easy way of life was to simply avoid overcrowding.

As the Industrial Revolution took hold, the days of the cottage industry and agrarian living would begin to slip away and would be another major factor in the migration. It was the story of new opportunity and greater wealth in these urban centers that would fuel the shift. From the earlier statistics, it is easy to see the growth of industry and population in bustling port cities.

Early immigrants were not afraid to take a chance on capitalizing on this growth and truly risk everything. They had the option of staying in their home lands where they knew the language, their past, and easily their future. But, this unknown and uncharted land across the Atlantic offered limitless possibilities no matter how bleak the odds of success were.

And how bleak were these odds of success and a better life? Let us examine the life of a poor farmer in Germany who decides he is going to take the chance in this new land.

First, how much money can this farmer raise by selling all his worldly possessions to fund this endeavor? Often very little if he was in a poor community with no one to sell his farm and equipment to. People prior to the Industrial Revolution would make their own tools and use them until they could not be used anymore – making selling even harder. For many, their greatest asset would be their offspring and family surrounding them with little worldly wealth to count. Many immigrants during the days of Ellis Island were successfully able to obtain steerage tickets either through selling whatever they knew they could not bring on their voyage or through families already in the United States, if they were lucky. Left with very little, these immigrants had no margin for error. This was compounded by the possibility that voyages could experience delay or take longer because of bad weather. Many immigrants would even be left without sufficient money to complete the entire voyage consisting of several legs in different ports.

To combat the risk, many immigrants were known to have sewn whatever excess cash they had left into the seams of their clothes for safe keeping on the journey. This was to avoid the temptation of gambling it away during the down times and to make sure there was something in safe keeping when packed into tight quarters.

Another great challenge would be for the farmer to safely arrive after his voyage across the Atlantic Ocean. Estimates are that nearly "three million shipwrecks lie on the ocean floor" spanning the history of man.[14] Not a very pleasant thought when being blown around in a sailing ship at sea in the early days of immigration.

With the rolling waves and the sheer uncertainty of conditions at different times of the year, the voyage could be brutal. Down in the steerage of the vessel, immigrants would be in tight quarters with limited food supply and fresh water. Disease would run rampant and the rising and falling seas would not make the voyage any more enjoyable. With hatches closed during bad weather, fresh air would be a dream come true when they would finally make it to land.

But alas, a farmer from Europe finally lays eyes on a distant shore in sight. With a skilled captain navigating, hopefully this sight is the correct destination if the winds cooperated. He has survived thus far and the thought of dry land under his feet in his only pair of shoes is an answered prayer. However, the real challenges are only about to begin for this new immigrant.

Arrival into one of the port cities, this young man would need to use whatever monetary resources he had left after paying for his voyage. If he was not fortunate enough to already have family in this new land, he would, in many cases, follow the language for a warm bed and meal. Just as Samuel Ellis would open a tavern on the remote Ellis Island, these meeting houses would be scattered through the bustling cities with many frequented by immigrants of the same country and language. These would prove to be valuable meeting points for one to find steady work, lodging and of course a celebratory drink for making it safely to America.

For the German immigrant, his next step would be to find steady employment which perhaps could be on the ever-expanding railroad or growing factory operations. This man would be well accustomed to brutally hard work and painful sacrifice. But how far would he go to survive in this land of opportunity?

According to an 1855 publication in Pittsburgh, "Railway brakemen had a life span that ended on average at 27, according to statistics published in The Daily Pittsburgh Gazette's June 19 edition."[15] The article would be spun though and note that only the "young and active men were employed in that capacity" which would mean that no one was going to stay in that space long enough to get killed like the employee before them. But if this farmer from Germany really wanted a full life in America, he would be wise to look into the service sector! The article notes that "Bakers died at 43 and butchers at 49, according to the Gazette story. Barbers lasted another full year, showing 'the virtue there is in personal neatness and soap and water.'"[15]

The money may prove good and perhaps he would be able to bring his family here to live a better life. The sacrifice of this one man would perhaps allow for future generations to know this land and live the promised life in America.

The famous story from Ellis Island is told that many immigrants believed they were going to be seeing 'streets paved in gold in America.' However, legend has it that one immigrant reflected on this with tongue and cheek humor. He noted that when he arrived, the streets were certainly not paved in gold and, in fact, not many streets were even paved at all! However, he was in shock to find that he could get paid to pave these streets for the very first time.

The American dream was worth chasing, but as Will Rogers would joke, "[e]ven if you're on the right track, you'll get run over if you just sit there." What remarkable risks these young immigrants took as they entered this new land and would refuse to stand idle in their quest for a better life.

CHAPTER 3: ENTERING THE CASTLE

> "Pleasure is a shadow, wealth is vanity, and power a pageant; but knowledge is ecstatic in enjoyment, perennial in frame, unlimited in space and indefinite in duration."
>
> – DeWitt Clinton

The first formal immigration center at New York would not be the Island of our story. It would be that of Castle Clinton at the foot of Manhattan, the dominating circle sandstone fort built as a harbor defense to stand alongside Fort Columbus, Fort Wood, and Fort Gibson. Castle Clinton would be the center of the forts securing the harbor and perhaps the key to the bastion in case of attack. The threat being prepared for was the brewing War of 1812 in case the British would try and attack New York. "The fort was fully armed with 28 cannons. Each cannon could shoot a 32 pound cannonball a distance of 1.5 miles," giving security to Manhattan as the center of New York and its commerce.16

As Castle Clinton, known during the War as 'Southwest Battery,' never had to fire on the enemy, it would be turned from a battle-ready fort to an entertainment hub for the growing city in 1823. Here, they would showcase opera, theatre, and even the famed Jenny Lind, the 'Swedish Nightingale,' brought to America by P.T. Barnum in 1850 to dazzle young and old audiences.

However, as immigration policy began to change in America, Castle Clinton would be eyed for the new beginning of the processing of a much-needed workforce to support the region.

As America emerged from the War of 1812 and stability began to reign, the land of liberty and opportunity would begin to grow at the seams. The Census issued during the summer of 1790 would count 3.9 million residents in the United States with a population of 4.5 people per square mile across thirteen states. Only thirty years later, in 1820, we would see a drastically different country on the rise. The population of nearly 10 million had spread itself across twenty-three states and had neighbors closer by, with 7.4 people occupying every square mile.[17]

The young federal government would continue to have fears with unbridled growth of the population spreading across the land. It would understand the need for a healthy country to enjoy prosperity after facing disease and epidemics from previous decades.

As the 19th century would see economic growth all around the world, shipping companies were seeing steady business of exporting goods such as cotton, lumber, and tobacco from the newly-formed United States. To improve profits though, they quickly realized they could have two-way traffic. Thus, on their voyage back to the new world, they would make use of their cargo holds to carry immigrants eager to work in these new industries in the United States.

This new business, however, caused an influx of unhealthy and poorly-treated immigrants who would be crammed into the steerage class section of the vessel on their journey to America. Their accommodation there was made up of no more than "wooden beds, known as berths, stacked two- to three-high with two people sharing single berths and up to four squeezed into a double."[18] To make matters worse in these cramped conditions, fresh air was limited below deck. Ventilation would be provided via hatches to the upper levels but was often locked during rough seas.

The state of poor immigrants, who often came from rural communities where they have not seen many contagious diseases, packed in together proved to be fatal once an outbreak occurred. Cleanliness options would be non-existent and the limited supply of fresh water and food made matters even worse. The new nation realized they had to try and improve the situation for these new immigrants or face deadly outbreaks in major cities which was so common of the era.

Thus, to bring a sense of order to this chaotic business, and recognizing from early colonial medicine that the spread of epidemics was best treated by providing a healthy diet and adequate space and hygiene, the fifteenth congress would enact the Steerage Act of 1819. The Act required that starting on the first day of 1820, a ship could carry no more than two persons for every five tons of vessel burden in accordance to customhouse measurement. The fine for breaking the Act was $150 for each person over the limit (over $3,500 today). The Act also required these companies to compile a ship manifest providing information of those onboard. The effort was effective not only in improving the damp, dark compartments that many immigrants were being subjected to, but also in making the companies accountable therefor. It was a first step to improve the dismal condition of those packed into the steerage class - if only to make their voyage, characterized by delays and violent seas less awful.

The United States would learn that a cramped ship being too tight and being a breeding ground for disease was not the only concern when dealing with immigration. As detailed in *The Greatest Benefit to Mankind*, Roy Porter details how Ireland set the table for understanding the health of new immigrants.

Ireland was a quickly growing country much like the United States. Being a small island nation, it was very densely populated. Relying on a staple crop of potato, they fell dependent on a steady food supply. However, "when the oat and potato crops failed, starving peasants became prey to various disorders, notably typhus, predictably called 'Irish fever' by the landlords."[19] The deadly outbreak of typhus and scurvy drove those who did not perish to look to immigrate.

However, Porter also notes that the Industrial Revolution encouraging this immigration may have had a worse trade-off. "While facilitating population growth and greater (if unequally distributed) prosperity, industrialization spread insanitary living conditions, workplace illnesses and 'new diseases' like rickets."[19] Rickets disease, caused by a vitamin D deficiency, would cause softening of bones, including delayed and malformed growth. Rickets would be most traumatic in children who could be working long laborious days in factories and mines of the mid-19th century.

As the 19th century progressed and the Industrial Revolution roared on, the demand for a strong working class grew. Even the Civil War would not drive away the demand. The demand for railroad construction, feeding, and clothing the feuding armies would not dissuade those hungry for the American dream. However, during the decades post the nation nearly being torn apart, Congress would work with the states to attempt to enhance regulations on immigration and make it a safer process.

The Immigration Act of 1882 would lay out even more unique standards aside from the general health of those in steerage class. USCIS (U.S. Citizenship and Immigration Services) notes that "the Chinese Exclusion Act of 1882 and Alien Contract Labor laws of 1885 and 1887 prohibited certain laborers from immigrating to the United States. The general Immigration Act of 1882 levied a head tax of fifty cents on each immigrant and blocked (or excluded) the entry of idiots, lunatics, convicts, and persons likely to become a public charge."[20] These harsh terms, which would be used for decades in the immigration process, were never clearly defined. Although it was clear that it was an early effort to make sure those entering the country were limited to the healthy and well.

So how did the port of New York in the United States fair as point of entry during all these years? During the period of 1855 to 1890, over eight million people entered the United States through Castle Clinton which would later be renamed as

Castle Garden. This castle though would be the beginning of formal immigration to New York.

However, as immigration continued to increase in the expanding nation, New York would look to formalize the process even more. Castle Garden would quickly change from an entertainment center to an immigration processing center on a warm summer day in 1855. With this being the first official emigrant landing depot, two out of every three immigrants to the United States in this period passed through this center and would have a story to tell.

As immigrants made the difficult decision to embark on this American journey or simply to escape war, famine, and disease in their home country, the view of coming into the New York harbor would have been a sight for sore eyes. However, with still little to no strict immigration process in place, getting through the door often came down to having the funds and willingness to work.

Before coming in to dock, a member of the boarding department would meet every vessel carrying the immigrants offshore. The officer would do an initial inspection of the vessel, record illness or death on board, and determine further navigation to the port.

If cleared, the vessel would be allowed to come

in to dock. Then the landing department would take over, with the Inspector of Customs overseeing the landing process. Luggage, if any, would be noted and reviewed and a quick medical inspection of the immigrants would commence. During the landing, a medical officer would conduct a visual examination of the immigrants to determine if any of them had a noticeable disease and would require quarantine offshore or if any of them are 'unfit' to work in the United States and, thus, posing a 'public charge.'

Once inside Castle Garden, registration could finally begin with the review of paperwork detailing an immigrant's name, nationality and intended destination. If no issues were found, an immigrant could then proceed out to what was believed was the American dream.

But not so fast! The South Street Sea Port Museum located in lower Manhattan detailed what lay in store. "Castle Garden became notorious for the solicitors and 'sharpers' who waited outside to take advantage of newcomers."[20] With demand for labor to build the rapidly growing city, need to build massive bridges such as the Brooklyn Bridge in 1869, and support the budding factories, labor bosses would post agents near the center to get first dibs on these poor new immigrants. With promise of 'good' pay and a warm bed, this would be a welcome offer.

To combat this issue of new immigrants being taken advantage of in New York City, "in 1873, to make sure immigrants could safely get to the New Jersey rail terminals, the Erie Railway negotiated a contract to run a ferry directly from Castle Garden."[21] This ferryboat contract would be a huge boost to the railroad company's growing business, allowing immigrants to travel and further their quest across the budding nation.

In Castle Garden, the immigrants were not able to exchange their currency. Outside, there were people waiting in dimly-lit corners looking to exchange money with the immigrants much higher than the market rate. Informational resources were also made available from a detailed pamphlet, albeit in proper English for those who were literate enough to read it.

The pamphlet entitled *Immigration and the Commissioners of Emigration of the State of New York* was put together by Friedrich Kapp, who was a Commissioner of Immigration at the site. The most interesting portion would be the support provided in assisting immigrants in obtaining a fair wage. In 1869, wages would range from $6 to $14 a month for a baker and $20 a month for cheese makers in accordance with the recommendation. However, "the wages for common laborers varied from $1.75 to $2 per day without board" in New York City in 1869.[22] This would come to just over $41 a day today – surely not going to get you very far in New York

City.

With the visions of the glitz, glamour, and bright lights of New York City's Time Square in mind today, the city of the late 1800's was filled with even more drive and grit in the hope of making it in this new world. With immigrants flooding into tenement housing in the Lower East Side of Manhattan, languages, foods, holidays, and lifestyles would be different all around.

Countless tales of immigrants crowding into small rooms to sleep on stiff bunks stacked to the ceilings with limited heat in the winter and poor ventilation in the summers was common place. This would make it even more difficult to rest after working often twelve-hour days, six days a week. Women who were often not able to enter the workforce, but were forced to raise children too young to work, would do their very best to keep these living arrangements clean. However, disease would often be an issue despite best efforts.

With low pay, immigrants' diets would only marginally improve here in the United States. The 'Garden State' of New Jersey and farms on Long Island would try and keep pace with providing fresh vegetables and unspoiled meats to the noisy street markets. Pasteurizing milk, something we take for granted today, would not even be a requirement in New York City until 1914. This mandate was implemented after a deadly outbreak of typhoid from contaminated raw milk containing salmonella bacterium.

The immigrants walking out from the musty Castle Garden into the blazing sun of New York's battery park may have felt like they were about to embark on the American dream. However, the challenges they faced and overcame should continue to make us thankful today. They were broken by the mountains they climbed just so future generations could prosper.

The move from Castle Garden to Ellis Island will take us across the sprawling harbor from the hustle and bustle of New York City to an island that would become just as famous and as filled with amazing history.

APPENDIX. 239

II.—*Wages paid for Skilled Labor in New York City during the Year 1869.*

Apprentices	$4 to $5 per week ; no board.
Bakers	$9 to $14 per month, and board.
Barbers	$9 to $15 per week ; no board.
Brushmakers	$2 to $2.50 per day ; no board.
Barkeepers	$10 to $30 per month, and board.
Basketmakers	$8 to $15 per week ; no board.
Blacksmiths	$2 to $5.50 per day ; no board.
Bookbinders	$7 to $18 per week ; no board.
Bricklayers	$5 per day ; no board.
Brewers	$15 to $25 per month, and board.
Brassfinishers	$10 to $20 per week ; no board.
Butchers	$10 to $30 per month, and board.
Cabinetmakers	$1.50 to $3 per day , no board.
Cooks	$25 to $100 per month, and board.
Capmakers	$8 to $12 per week, and board.
Chemists	$10 to $12 per week ; no board.
Carpenters	$3 to $3.50 per day ; no board.
Carriagemakers	$2.50 to $3 per day ; no board.
Cheesemakers	$20 per month, and board.
Cigarmakers	$8 to $15 per week ; no board.
Confectioners	$30 to $50 per month, and board.
Cutlers	$12 to $15 per week , no board.
Coopers	$18 to $20 per week ; no board.
Dyers	$20 to $25 per month, and board.
Dockhands	$25 to $30 per month, and board.
Druggists	$18 to $35 per month, and board
Engravers	$15 to $35 per week ; no board.
Engineers	$15 to $18 per week ; no board.
Florists	$15 to $35 per month, and board
Filecutters	$12 to $18 per week ; no board.
Furriers	$9 to $14 per week ; no board.
Fresco-painters	$15 to $35 per week ; no board.
Gilders	$10 to $18 per week ; no board.
Gardeners	$15 to $25 per month, and board.
Glaziers	$8 to $12 per week ; no board.
Gasfitters	$12 to $18 per week ; no board.
Goldsmiths	$10 to $30 per week ; no board.
Gunsmiths	$10 to $18 per week ; no board.
Hatters	$15 to $20 per week ; no board.
Heaters	$25 to $30 per month, and board
Harnessmakers	$10 to $15 per week ; no board.
Ironmoulders	$15 to $18 per week ; no board.
Locksmiths	$8 to $15 per week ; no board.
Lithographers	$12 to $25 per week ; no board.
Machinists	$15 to $18 per week ; no board.

Wage expectations for an immigrant in New York City in 1869

Kapp, Friedrich. Immigration, and the Commissioners of Emigration of the State of New York. Gale, Sabin Americana, 2012.

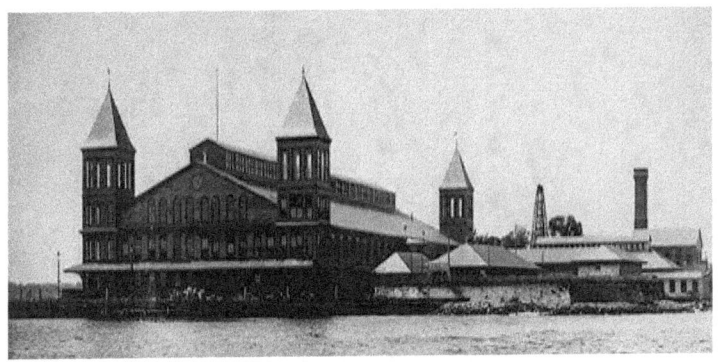

(above) The original immigration station c. 1892-1897

National Archives and Records Administration

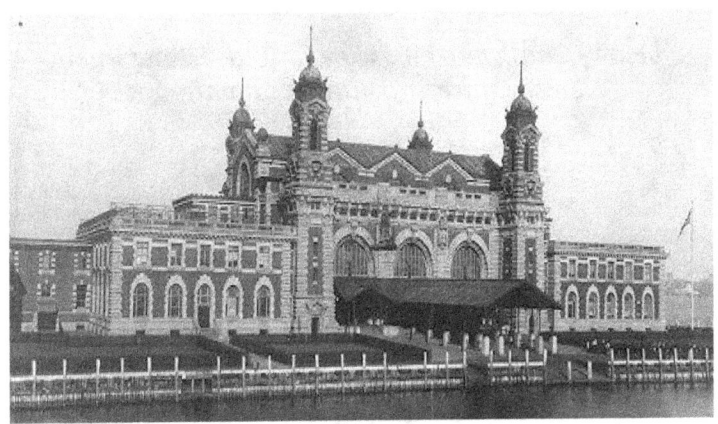

(above) The newly built Main Immigration Building c.1904 - 1910.

National Archives and Records Administration

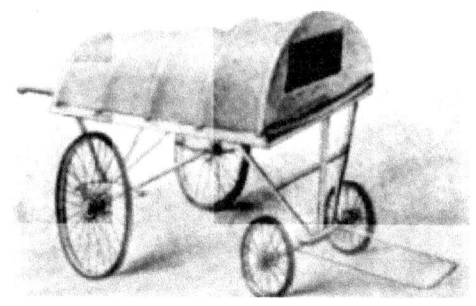

(above) Drawing of 'hand ambulance' for transporting patients through the Contagious Disease Hospital at Ellis Island

The Modern Hospital. July 1917 ed., IX, McGraw-Hill. (pg. 316).

(below) Chalk markings key for Ellis Island Public Health Officers to mark on immigrants

X – Suspected Mental Defect
Ⓧ – Definite Mental Defect
B – Back
E – Eyes
F – Face
Ft – Feet
G – Goiter
H – Heart
K – Hernia
L – Lameness
LWF – Landed with Fever
N – Neck
P – Physical & Lungs
Pg – Pregnant
SC – Scalp (Favus)

HAD ELLIS ISLAND WASHED AWAY

View of General Health Hospital from Island 1 today

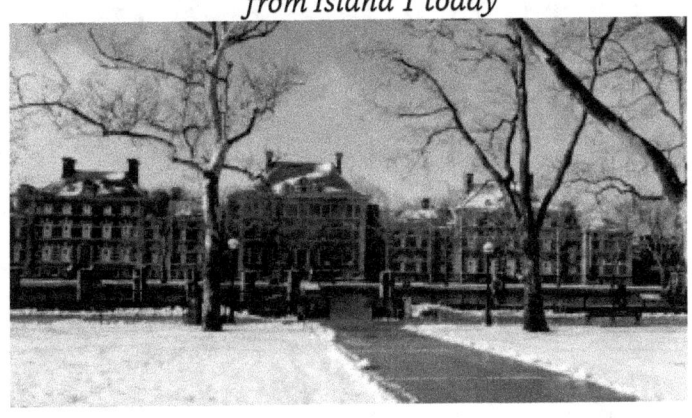

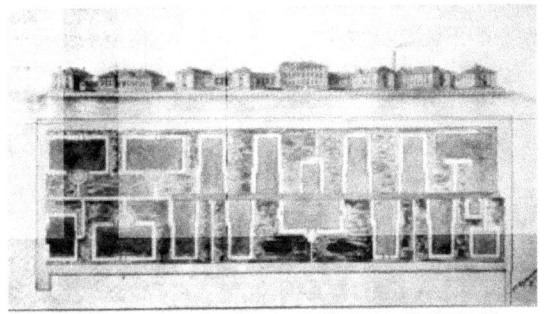

Fig. 1. View and ground floor plan of the Contagious Disease Hospital for Immigrants at Ellis Island, New York.

View and ground floor plan of Contagious Disease Hospital at Ellis Island

The Modern Hospital. July 1917 ed., IX, McGraw-Hill. (p 316).

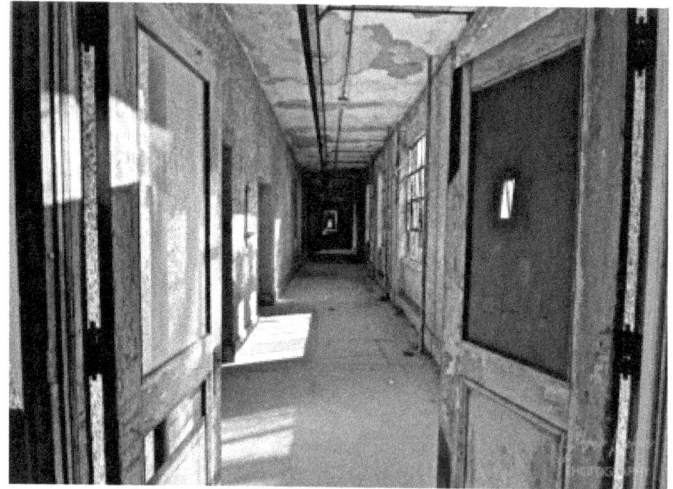

(above) Hall of Contagious Disease Hospital today (Island 3)
– Courtesy, Shane Kiefer Photography

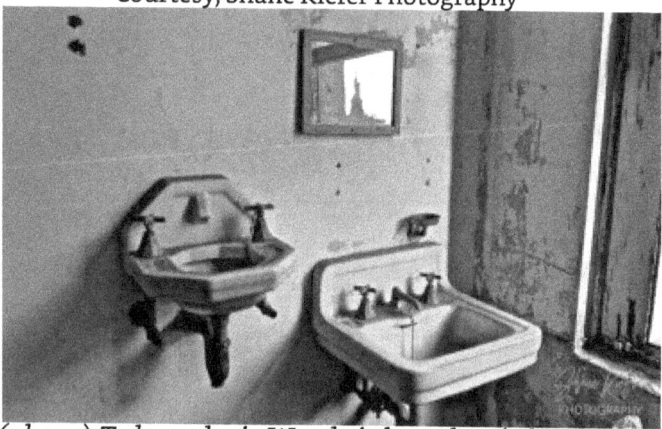

(above) Tuberculosis Ward sinks today (Island 3)
– Courtesy, Shane Kiefer Photography

PART II: THE BEGINNINGS OF ELLIS ISLAND

CHAPTER 4: OYSTER ISLAND TO ELLIS ISLAND

> "We must not forget that these men and women who file through the narrow gates at Ellis Island, hopeful, confused, with bundles of misconceptions as heavy as the great sacks upon their backs these simple, rough-handed people are the ancestors of our descendants, the fathers and mothers of our children."
>
> – Walter Weyl

On a beautiful sunny afternoon, as you rowed out towards Ellis Island prior to 1892, you would see a crumbling fort and the large supplies of powder magazines stored by the US Navy. There was very little activity for an island guarding the harbor. Soon, however, it would be the island welcoming those from abroad for the very first time.

With the nation continuing its compounding growth out of the Industrial Revolution and post-Civil War expansion, the federal government would step in and take responsibility from the states on the regulation and processing of immigration.

The Immigration Act of 1891 was built on previous pieces of government legislation regulating the growing number of immigrants sailing for the United States. The Act would impose a head tax per immigrant and would require documentation of their biographical information by the shipping company (in the form of an enhanced manifest). However, no matter how noble the purposes of the Act were, it created bureaucracy in the form of the Office of Superintendent of Immigration. The head of this office, appointed by the President of the United States, would fall under the jurisdiction of the Secretary of the Treasury and would oversee the growing number of immigration inspectors stationed at the ports. The Act, unfortunately, would also extend for ten more years the Chinese Exclusion Act which was first put in place 1882 to prohibit the immigration of Chinese laborers.

With this new Act in place, government funds were appropriated to build a brand new immigration station off of the island of Manhattan for the first time. Ellis Island would give quick and easy access to the large ships docking in New York, as well as provide quarantine location for those who contracted disease onboard the large ships.

"On May 24, 1890, the federal government formally transferred Ellis Island from the War Department to the Department of the Treasury," who was now placed in charge of immigration.[23]

Construction would quickly begin on Ellis Island after it was expanded from three acres to six acres via landfill in the choppy forty-foot waters around the island. With a proper ferry slip constructed, and beautiful three-story Georgia pine immigration processing center in the middle of Ellis Island finally in place, immigration would commence on January 1, 1892.

With seventeen year old Annie Moore of Ireland stepping off the SS Nevada to board a ferry for Ellis Island, the legacy of the Island would begin. Eleven days prior, on December 20th, she would leave behind her home of Ireland to begin her new life in America. As with many immigrants, her parents and older siblings had already made the voyage to America to begin saving up to bring the rest of the family to this new land one day. She would make the voyage with her two younger brothers as her escort.

Arriving late on December 31st, Annie's ship would lay at anchor until the morning of New Year's Day. "At 10:30 a.m. on New Year's Day, a flag on Ellis Island was dipped three times as a signal to transport the first boatload of immigrants."[24] With surrounding ships joining in the joy with clanging bells and chirping whistles, the first ferry of steerage class passengers would cross the chilly harbor for processing. Decked out in red, white, and blue banners, the ferry would glide into the dock at Ellis.

As Annie entered the center, she would make her way easily up the main steps to the famous registry room. Charles Hendley would have the honor of being the first Treasury Department official to register Annie. With a quick stroke of the pen, the review of Annie's manifest would be completed. Annie would then be met by former congressman John B. Weber who had assumed the role of Superintendent of Immigration for the Port of New York. Mr. Weber would greet Annie and gently place in her hand a ten-dollar gold piece in honor of her being the first immigrant to complete the processing. On the day that Annie arrived, nearly 700 more immigrants came and experienced the newly-inaugurated center.

As Annie walked out of the center, she would then be greeted and embraced by the parents she had not seen in years. She would be swiftly taken onto a ferry from Ellis Island to the hustle and bustle of Manhattan to finally be able to put her feet firmly in this new land. She would live the American dream, as it was viewed, albeit it was a hard life living in the Lower East Side of Manhattan. Marrying a German-American, she would have

10 children according to records, with only "five surviving to adulthood" according to a 2006 New York Times article of her life.[25] Annie would pass in 1924 at the age of 50, although her legacy would be remembered in the halls of Ellis Island and Ireland to this day.

With the economy slowing in the last decade of the 1800's, immigration was often slow at Ellis Island. With fewer than 20,000 eager immigrants using the center each year, it was seldom overwhelmed. After five years of use, a fire would rip through the wooden center on the morning of June 15, 1897 destroying the handsome buildings on site. With the quick action of those on hand, thankfully, no one would be killed. Immigration would move back to a barge office in Battery Park while the government partnered with the New York architectural firm of Boring and Tilton to build a new fireproof center on Ellis Island to serve the next wave of immigrants to come.

As the new century dawned, and hopes of improving economies globally grew, the new immigration center would open on December 17, 1900. The beautifully ornate new center was skillfully constructed in the Beaux-Arts Classical design. Many of the laborers were from previous waves of immigrants who willingly built the new gateway for future generations to pass through.

The new center would even be a first of its

kind, being built with strong fireproof limestone and brick as the main components. This would allow standing the test of time and harsh harbor storms. With large windows on all sides, light could dance across the room with no obstruction from the harbor. The beautiful main registration room on the second floor would utilize the Guastavino Fireproof Construction Company to install their patented interlocking tiles to ornate the tall vaulted ceiling.

The main room would also have drains installed all throughout and fire hoses on each wall. While this was a great resource in case of fire, this would serve another purpose. At that time, there was no air conditioning and only the ocean breeze was there to cool off hundreds of anxious immigrants in heavy wool suits. After a day of sweating, and after a long voyage with likely no bath, the center would be hosed down to prepare it for the following day's wave of inspections.

With the beautiful new center opened, the Island would see an ever-growing influx of eager immigrants which would peak only a few short years later in 1907. In this one year alone, Ellis Island would see over one million immigrants enter the nation via its doors.

Immigrants would hail from all over Europe and the largest populations of steerage class passengers came in the early part of the 20th century from Ireland, Germany, and Italy. These immigrants with calloused hands, weather-worn clothes, and a big dream would be the backbone of the growing economy. With larger and larger ships entering the harbor, the process of screening would have to keep up.

With an initial quarantine stop off the southern tip of Staten Island before entering the harbor, a ship would be quickly checked over by a group of immigration inspectors for any outbreak of contagious disease. If all clear, the ship could continue into the harbor to dock along the Hudson or East River, depending on the assigned dock for the shipping company. From there, the first- and second-class passengers could disembark with relative ease after a review by bureau staff onboard the ship. These were the individuals who had the money and resources in life. Businessmen, industrialists, doctors, and lawyers would go through a simple questioning and off they went.

However, half the vessel (which could be in the thousands) would be made up of the third-class passengers also known as the steerage class. These were the individuals who would need to be ferried to Ellis Island for further questioning and proper medical exam. Confronted by burly immigration inspectors, their small worn bags would be checked for any illegal contraband or smuggled goods. They would then be tagged with a tan-colored manifest tag to be ferried off to Ellis Island for further questioning.

Boarding a small white ferryboat operated by the Department of Treasury, the journey by sea would continue from the island they may have hoped to call home to the famous Ellis Island. It would be on this island that the decision on their fate and future would be made.

As the ferryboat coasted into the slip at Ellis Island, the large opposing building would be their first home in America for the next three to five hours assuming no problems arose. These would be tense hours of walking in line, watching for steely glances from healthy and strong Americans in military uniforms, and waiting on stiff wooden benches. With many only having literacy in their mother tongue, the commands in another language would make the process even scarier. Thankfully, translators were available and inspectors and doctors would often be able to speak in multiple languages, making the process smoother and less stressful.

One well known interpreter would be a second generation American and young law student from New York City, Fiorello H. La Guardia. La Guardia would work for the Bureau of Immigration on the Island and was fluent in Italian, Yiddish, and Croatian. It was likely not a bad place to meet constituents for his future mayoral campaign. It is ironic to note that an airport in his name, LaGuardia International, does not have Customs and Border Protection facilities today driving many international arrivals to John F. Kennedy International Airport in New York. Interesting to ponder what he would have thought of that?

But decades before flights would bring immigrants into the nation, inspectors and interpreters like La Guardia would be the welcoming committee. As immigrants' names would be called, echoing throughout the second floor of the Great Hall, they would approach the inspectors at the front of the room towards the western side. The inspectors would be perched behind large wooden desks with a team of translators working amongst them for difficult or unknown dialects. With manifests in the hands of the inspectors, the immigrants would be asked to confirm their information and answer some questions.

The inspectors would review the manifest which contained a series of roughly twenty questions varying over the years. Details included nationality, height, hair color, and even the amount of money on hand. From here, the inspectors may have questions ranging from work experience and family resources. Much of this was to confirm authenticity and accuracy of information provided regarding background and intention for migrating. With the dash of a pen, the interview could be over in a flash if no issues arose.

One of the unique questions though that often added potential for slip ups was added to the manifest as part of the Immigration Act of 1903. With the tragic assassination of President William McKinley in September of 1901 by a self-proclaimed anarchist, the question of whether one is an anarchist would be added to the manifest in an effort to prevent this evil ideology from entering the nation. Stories go that during the interview, the inspector would re-read this question which was believed to be answerable with a simple response. Legend goes, however, that if you answered too quickly with a 'No,' glanced away during your response, or even paused, you would be further asked how you even knew what that word meant.

For those who may have had a questionable past, or were caught in lies, the only option for them would be what was called the Board of Special Inquiry, a court-like system on Ellis Island. The immigrants would be removed from processing and a new dormitory space on the Island would have to be their temporary home. The most common violation these immigrants faced was that of being "a likely public charge on economic or medical grounds."[26] This could be assumed by the inspectors on grounds that they had a fear that the immigrant standing before them may be unable or unwilling to support oneself upon entry to the country.

Often through appearing before the Board and demonstrating a willingness to work and support their families, immigrants could obtain approval from the Board and make it through processing in a few short days. The Board process, however, was not often easy as immigrants would have to plead their case in broken language and with great strain knowing that their lives and the lives of their families depended on the outcome of this hearing.

For many of these immigrants, the Board hearing would be a plea for life and a future. This is because, at this point, all they had left in life would only fill a small trunk. With their Sunday best on their back, and perhaps two sets of weathered work clothes, many would be carrying their family bible. These bibles would be well-worn from past generations who held strongly to their faith and found encouragement from John 10:10 which says that "I have come that they might have life, and that they might have it more abundantly." Indeed, their plea during this hearing was not for a career in America, but to be given a chance to at least start a new life in this nation with the hope that they can fulfill His will in their lives here.

If all could go well though for the immigrant, they would have the joy of descending what was called the stairs of separation. To be greeted by family waiting for them, to make it through with the whole family, and to be deemed healthy enough to figure out where to begin their journey in this new land would be a dream enough at the bottom of the staircase.

The factor of separation at the stairs was more

a fear if one or multiple members of the family would be deemed 'unfit' to enter the country. This was often rare as only two percent of all immigrants were sent back to their home country. However, in reality, that is nearly a third of a million people who did not get to go down the stairs to begin their journey - lives that would not get to live the American dream. These were grandparents too weak to work hard labor, children deathly-ill with a contagious disease, and groups of single women fleeing abuse back home.

Families would have to make the extremely difficult decision of who may stay or go as children would have to be accompanied home. Able bodied men and boys would often get priority to stay in the country to put in the arduous work to try again to reunite the family at a future date and time. This could be years away for many and, for some, the time would never come. The journey across the ocean was no guarantee - a fact never to be overlooked.

For ninety percent of the immigrants who made their way through the process, the three to five hours of questioning in the Great Hall would be all they knew and remembered of Ellis Island. The greatest memory for many would be making their way out of the immigration center, but not before stopping at the bottom of the stairs at what would be remembered as the 'kissing post' - a place for families to finally breathe a sigh of relief, feel the overwhelming joy of what would lay ahead, and either kiss each other or the ground of the nation that allowed them to enter its doors.

However, for those who were not so fortunate in those hours on site and had gotten sick onboard the vessel to the United States, Ellis Island would grow to offer more to support their desire at a fair chance at the American dream.

The Island would have to develop its footprint even larger from the early decade of use to meet the influx of immigrants to the United States. Ellis Island would grow ever larger with landfill additions over the years to accommodate additions of a sprawling kitchen, laundry facility and onsite powerplant. The greatest additions would be in the form of state-of-the-art hospitals.

The demand for growth was not necessarily because of the interview and inspection process within the Great Hall as, prior to the 1920's in America, there was neither paper passport nor visa to hold up the process. The real demand was because of the necessity to ensure that these new immigrants were healthy and ready to work – work harder than they ever dreamed for the American dream they wanted to hold so dearly in their grasp. Thus, the expansion of the hospital complex at Ellis Island.

CHAPTER 5: ABLE BODIED WORKERS

"I will remember that I do not treat a fever chart, a cancerous growth, but a sick human being, whose illness may affect the person's family and economic stability. My responsibility includes these related problems, if I am to care adequately for the sick..."

– Hippocratic Oath excerpt

As shadows grow long across the red brickwork floor of the Great Hall at Ellis Island, a group of young immigrants shuffle forward in their only set of shoes towards an imposing American in military dress. The man is a doctor working for the United States Public Health Service whose mission is to protect the general health and wellbeing of the public. In his dress blues, he appears ready to command an army with any weapon he holds. However, his weapon of choice today is a tiny tool called a buttonhook. This tiny instrument, along with his eyes, will be his weapons in a quest to literally preserve these immigrants' own eyes and secure their futures in this new land.

Alongside him are practitioners who would become the forefront of modern medicine in America, supporting public health around the world. They would be pioneers in their work and would even be one of the first doctors that many immigrants would ever see in their whole lives as they embarked on their journey in America.

Their name would change over the years but their commitment to promoting the general health would not waver. As the new nation was just being created, the Public Health Service would be known as the Marine Hospital Fund beginning in 1798. That was nearly a century before Ellis Island would see them at work.

President John Adams, more than anyone else, would understand the need to protect the public health. As the pioneering champion of the United States Navy during his extensive Revolutionary War travels, he had a fair share of witnessing outbreaks of disease in his lifetime. He came to the correct conclusion that public health was greatly impacted by the travel of goods and services. His solution was to protect the public through "An Act for the relief of sick and disabled Seamen" who may be transporting disease in addition to the cargos.[27]

Early healthcare in America was more of a mystical art than a learned science. With the landing of the first settlers to America, they also landed with disease. Native populations would stand no chance to the likes of smallpox and typhus – diseases they have never seen before. With fevers breaking out from these deadly diseases, whole communities would be devastated and wiped out in a season.

One early example of a disease that repeatedly ravaged the colonies, small pox, would be seen in the growing port city of Boston in 1721. A doctor during that era would rise to the challenge of fighting this unseen enemy, Zabdiel Boylston.

Dr. Boylston was a son of a physician and was born in the new colony of Massachusetts in 1679. With no formal medical schooling to find for nearly a century, he would apprentice under his father and would later go on to challenge the previous standards of medicine.

Many physicians at that time followed well-known and accepted methods of treatments practiced over the centuries. These methods, which included quarantining the ill, bleeding and purging, were all thought to restore the body to its natural state and balance of health.

With another outbreak of smallpox beginning to ravage Boston in 1721, it would take the friendship between Reverend Cotton Mather, the pastor of the Congregationalist North Church of Boston, and Dr. Boylston to wage war against the disease. As many illnesses were seen as the work of the devil, the relationship between religion and medicine were deeply intertwined.

Mather, with his inquisitive mind, would find "articles in the Royal Society of London's *Philosophical Transaction* detailing a little-known Asian and Middle Eastern folk medicine practice of inoculation for small-pox."[28] On the other hand, Boylston experienced small-pox himself during his youth. He also accomplished many firsts in medicine such as first surgeries to remove gall bladder stones and breast tumor.

Together, Mather and Boylston would unite against many doubters to fight small-pox. With taking the puss and scabs from those currently infected, and placing the sample inside a small cut of a healthy patient, they would work to create immunity against future outbreaks. Their quest was not met without hostility and even threats of death. However, their new tool to fight disease would live on for future generations.

While the method of inoculation was challenged, its benefits were realized over the decades. During the Revolutionary War, General George Washington fought against the British's attempt to wage a 'biological warfare' by sending sick refugees into the Continental Army camps to spread disease to tired American troops. Washington implemented standards of inoculation and hygiene in camps, helping Americans fight back on all fronts.

Early hospitals were also a foreign idea to many. With the founding of Bellevue Hospital in 1736 and the Pennsylvania Hospital in the 1751, these early institutions were more of a place to go and die rather than a place to seek treatment and cure. The early hospitals lacked formal training, sanitation, and were often only used as a last resort.

By the 19th century, President Adams planted the seeds of modern medicine as he established the Marine Hospital Fund under the control of the United States Treasury Department. The fund would require customs to be collected from each sailor to fund a hospital service for their care.

As more formal training for new doctors, surgeons, and nurses would evolve during the early part of the 19th century, disease would still pose a threat to an ever-growing country. As the nation would be nearly torn apart by civil war in 1861, a person born in the United States could hope to live a long life just short of forty years of age! This number had only marginally increased, although with more advanced training, transference of ideas and understanding, the medical profession was making strides.

With the nation coming out of the Industrial Revolution, and people now being more mobile via the expanding train lines, disease would also continue to spread.

The concern, however, was not only the domestic spread of sickness and disease, but also the threat from seagoing immigrants who were traveling in cramped, dirty, and tight quarters to the new world. In these often damp and dirty quarters, disease would thrive. For the medical personnel taking on the duty of working with the Public Health Service, they would be the first line of defense to making sure the general public remained healthy and well. To the layperson, the fear that immigrants may be carrying diseases is a battle we still face today.

The early practice of medical exam for the immigration process was to do a visual inspection of the vessel and speak to passengers and crew on any known outbreaks en route. If a vessel was known to have such an outbreak, the vessel would have to become a quarantine vessel if no room at the quarantine hospitals near and on Staten Island was available. The vessel would then need to remain at anchor in the harbor until the outbreak had ended which could be take months and countless healthy lives.

To combat the fear of citizens, the first quarantine facilities built in the Hudson River would be that of Swinburne Island in 1860 and Hoffman Island in 1873. These small manmade islands would offer a quick option to offboard sick passengers for quarantine although it did not always offer premier medical care.

As Ellis Island had just opened in 1892, the early medical center was to be put to the test. The two-story dispensary had limited supplies, beds, and experience with treating any type of epidemic.

During the summer of 1892, a cholera epidemic - one of many over the century - was crisscrossing Europe and Asia. As immigrants and refugees fled Europe, their hope of safety was soon to be challenged. As the first of what would be referred to as 'death ships' entered the harbor, the Moravia ship would be forced to contain over one thousand passengers who were stranded as no local hospitals had rooms or even willingness to take them in. Lorie Conway details in her book, *Forgotten Ellis Island*, that the scare would be documented in local newspapers and journals. "Their plea was denied, and over the next several days, additional cases broke out, killing most of the infected passengers. Not until nearly three weeks had passed were the healthy passengers finally allowed to disembark."[29]

As a number of vessels were bringing immigrants from Germany, the terrible and deadly cholera outbreaks continued sweeping across these death ships. As cholera was a waterborne disease, it would nearly all passengers across different classes would become deathly ill. With fears mounting of what to do with all the sick, these hospitals would be overwhelmed and not be able to keep pace. The greatest anger would rise from the public over hotels being used as hospitals and was met with violent opposition.

As the new modern immigration center was opening after being burnt in 1897, the debate about developing advanced, larger, and more hygienic hospitals was underway. As the new century began, President Theodore Roosevelt would outline what the future of healthcare for these immigrants would look like. As President Roosevelt prepared for his first State of the Union in December of 1901, he would outline a new immigration system, to wit:

> Our present immigration laws are unsatisfactory. We need every honest and efficient immigrant fitted to become an American citizen, every immigrant who comes here to stay, who brings here a strong body, a stout heart, a good head, and a resolute purpose to do his duty well in every way and to bring up his children as law-abiding and God-fearing members of the community.[30]

As President Roosevelt called upon the government to begin implementing new controls and procedures for the immigration service, he would also call on the Public Health Service in particular to make sure that America would be able to meet the rising demands thrust upon her. By putting more rigid controls on health on both sides of the wide ocean, they would perhaps be able to control the outbreak of diseases, as well as prepare hospitals to fight the challenges in the new century. By referring to an immigrant with a "strong body, a stout heart, and a good head," President Roosevelt called for an able and ready immigrant to see the opportunity in the nation.

At Ellis Island, work was already underway to meet this challenge in a way never imagined and in ways that still amaze visitors to the Island today.

The first hospital structure to be built at Ellis Island would begin on what would be referred to as Island 2. This Island, much like the greater part of Island 1, would be built using landfill from dredging operations in the shipping channels in the harbor. With only a narrow strip of dirt connecting southwards from Island 1 and the immigration center, Island 2 would be built much the same size. It would be filled in with landfill and rock with large limestone rocks and caissons being lowered into the waters. Island 2, a new man-made island, would house the first hospital post the fire.

At a cost of $33,000 in 1902 (just over $1,070,000 today), construction would begin. The goal was to build a hospital with the capacity of over 120 patient beds, and wards broken out by disease off an expansive central hall. It would provide space for surgeries to be conducted, delivery room for newborns, laboratories for testing, and a morgue for learning. The large dormer windows allowed in natural sunlight and fresh ocean breeze which helped promote hygiene and sanitation. Between the wards, a central hallway would run, expanding the footprint of the hospital from west to east and with beautiful mosaic tiling. For those who wanted even more of the beautiful views and sunlight, balconies would be constructed on the southern side of the hospital to take in the lovely harbor.

With grand open staircases made of dark slate reaching to the third floors to have quick access to patients. As a form of quarantine and quick access to patients, doctors and nurses would be housed right in the middle of the hospital. For those patients too sick to climb the stairs, the hospital would also operate an Otis Elevator to take patients to the upper floors where the operating rooms would be found.

In these operating rooms which had white subway tile wrapping from floor to ceiling, surgeons would be able to provide relief and recovery for men who had worked hard lives abroad and prepare them to work hard again. Performing surgeries for hernias would become a specialty. Directly over the operating room table would be a glass skylight with copper frame set into the red Spanish terracotta roof. Through this skylight, patients were able to look straight ahead to the beautiful blue sky as they lay on a cold metal table.

Not only was the skylight a wonderful addition for natural sunlight in the operating room, but it also served another key purpose. The use of ether in anesthesiology was the standard practice. Ether gas would rise into the air when administered to the patient which could waft out of the skylight when opened by a crank lever. This was also critical as ether, when mixed with oxygen, is highly combustible. Retaining ether in an operating room was a danger to all.

With immigration increasing at the turn of the century, the hospital would continue its growth towards the eastern edge of the new island it was built upon. It would even expand its services to treat the 'idiots' and 'imbeciles' which the immigration service was most worried about slipping into the country.

In opening up a psychopathic pavilion, Ellis Island would be a leader in treating mental health disorders as humanely as possible. However, the use of electroshock, hydrotherapy, and other rudimentary techniques were still the accepted practice of the era. Interestingly, hydrotherapy often involved soaking a patient in an ice bath. A patient who was experiencing high fever may have appeared to be going through a mental health episode. Inadvertently, the ice bath would bring the patient's internal body temperature back to a normal level. Today, a cage still protrudes from the hospital ward which gave immigrants outdoor space for fresh air if they found themselves in a state of shock after being considered a 'lunatic.'

As immigrants step down the wooden boardwalk at Ellis Island, they were haggard, tired, and scared. Surely, their mental state was not at its peak in the warm noonday sun. These immigrants who had just left everything behind were, in many cases, alone. They had just endured a difficult journey and had such fears of the unknown that lay ahead. Separated from loved ones, with no happy faces to welcome them, immigrants' minds would surely begin to race.

If a Public Health official would make the decision to pull them from line, it could be from a simple observation of the immigrant's demeanor. It could be for not making eye contact with a bowed head towards men in military uniform. For some, it may be the act of talking to oneself in line to prepare for the questions ahead. It would not be a surprise at all to deduce that this immigrant may not be ready to face the challenges that were ahead.

For many who would find themselves in the psychopathic pavilion, this would be a scary time. The hospital recognized that, at this state, it would be fruitless to have immigrants undergo questioning again immediately. Thus, to make the process more humane, many doctors would allow these scared immigrants to have a hot meal and good night's rest knowing that there was no good in working with the exhausted. After resting on a stable cotton mattress - as opposed to the swaying bunks in the bottom of a boat - many immigrants would in fact be in much better spirits to undergo another questioning. The hospital also discovered that it was more helpful to do the questioning before the Board of Special Inquiry, as opposed to the echoing noise in the Great Hall surrounded by hundreds of observers.

Mental health in America was certainly making great strides at Ellis Island and one would have to wonder if it was because of healthy food... or was there something in fact in the water?

Just to the northwest of Ellis Island was the ever-growing city of Jersey City, New Jersey. As a large port city with train lines coming in from all over the east coast, as well as a home for many new immigrants stretching up to Hoboken, this was a city on the rise. Dr. John L. Leal would join the East Jersey Water Company in 1899, after being a health officer for another growing nearby city, Paterson, New Jersey. Working as a sanitary advisor, he would look to improve water quality to the burgeoning communities they serviced.

With large cities having blurred lines between how sewage was being removed and how fresh water was being provided to residents, waterborne disease and epidemics were becoming more and more common. With Dr. Leal working with Jersey City on implementing a new reservoir system, Jersey City would become the first city in the nation to disinfect their water starting in 1908. According to the CDC, "over the next decade, thousands of cities and towns across the United States followed suit in routinely disinfecting their drinking water, contributing to a dramatic decrease in disease across the country."[31]

With pipes stretching from treatment centers in Jersey City, drinking water could now be piped out to Ellis Island. This would be a great improvement over the previously-installed rainwater cisterns which were exposed to the elements. The chance to give immigrants a taste of clean and fresh water for the very first time perhaps in their lives and after a rough trip at sea would be a godsend.

For many, it would feel like their lives were just beginning as they left Ellis Island. Indeed, for some, it truly was literally just the beginning as records note that 424 babies were born in the General Health Hospital of Ellis Island.

With woman coming through the immigration process and showing as 'noticeably pregnant,' they would be marked with 'PG' on the lapel of their jackets and escorted to the maternity ward in the General Health Hospital on Island 2. With the overwhelming majority of woman still giving birth at home at the turn of the 20th century, the opportunity to give birth in a hospital would drastically improve the chances of survival for a child. At the same time, it would decrease maternal mortality from complications which could be easily addressed with proper medical facilities and trained staff.

To go one step further in care, the Ellis Island hospitals would even have female physicians on staff – a rarity in hospitals around the world. For many women, it was a comfort to be examined by a female physician for the first time. To validate the success of this relationship, one of the most famous female physicians at Ellis Island, Dr. Rose Bebb, would advance to the staff of the psychiatric department of Bellevue Hospital. In the Surgeon General's Annual Report of 1914, it was noted that "for obvious reasons this measure has resulted in rendering practicable a more critical inspection of women immigrants turned aside for further medical examination and is regarded as making for increased efficiency."

To note though, thanks to the detailed records kept by the surgeon general, of the 1,387 physicians who would work and live on the Island over all the decades, only 38 of them were female. This would prove to be a lower percentile than that in private practice. Moreover, these female doctors never worked within the walls of the hospital. At that time, doctors at Ellis Island would be assigned to either work in the hospital or in the immigration processing line. Working in the hospitals would be considered the most prestigious and only the best of surgeons and physicians would make it there. Working in the immigration processing line, while as equally important, was considered less esteemed. Unfortunately for female doctors at that time, no matter how skilled they were, they would always be assigned to work in the line. This assignment, however, was partly due to the fact that the female doctors' focus then would be to confirm if an immigrant was pregnant upon arrival. As this would require disrobing in a separate room, female physicians would oversee the procedure, making it a much more humane process for immigrants going through the immigration line.

However, working for the Public Health Service truly set many of these female doctors up for leadership roles in their practice such as Dr. Bebb. Many of them had already achieved greatness in their profession and their time at Ellis Island would be the pinnacle of their careers in caring for their patients.

With immigration continuing its climactic rise, the bed count in the hospital on Island 2 would also need to rise. Growing up to 275 patient beds, it was seeing its resources stretched like never before.

The greater concern was also how to provide more space to avoid the spread of contagious diseases. The problems were further compounded with the need to separate patients by gender and ward.

As New York City continued to grow its shipping operations, additional dredged landfill of clay, sand, and gravel would be produced and would be used to support the physical expansion of Ellis Island. In an effort to deal with the mounting influx of patients, a new hospital would need to be constructed to deal solely with contagious diseases. This hospital would need to be on a scale like never seen before. The idea of having isolated contagious and infectious disease hospitals was not a new idea in America or the world.

Throughout history, the concept and treatment of those with infectious diseases would often simply involve undergoing quarantine. However, the idea of having immigrants undergo quarantine in a premier medical facility as a standard was as foreign as these immigrants were to the new nation.

Treating a disease regardless of race, religion, or gender was engrained in the Hippocratic Oath that all doctors had learned over millennia. But now they would be taking this to heart. During this time, the nation was indeed going through a rebirth as it strived to extend to immigrants one of the most fundamental aspirations of the Declaration of Independence, that is, the giving of 'unalienable rights of life, liberty, and the pursuit of happiness.' Perhaps it was not just in life, but in giving a 'healthy life' that liberty could finally be obtained for all who wanted to pursue it well. It was now up to the Public Health Service to face these diseases head on for the very first time.

CHAPTER 6: THE Y IN THE ROAD

"Fear of disease killed more men than disease itself."

– Mahatma Gandhi

The famous baseball player for the New York Yankees, Yogi Berra, once said in his sly sense of humor, "when you come to a fork in the road – take it!" That joyful sense of humor has always been a highlight on my hospital tours at Ellis Island as guests peer down the dark 'Y Corridor.'

The Y Corridor was a physical dividing line in the hospital complex located on Island 2 where one corridor leads to the General Health Hospital while the other one leads to the Contagious Disease Hospital. This point marks yet another chapter of battle that immigrants have to hurdle before they can begin their lives in America. Thankfully, many would carry with them that undying hope of seeing their families again whom they have bid goodbye just a few moments prior to reaching the Y Corridor. Located just a few yards before the Y Corridor was the Ferry Building where family members who had been cleared to leave would take the boat for New York or New Jersey. It was at this Ferry Building that the immigrants destined to traverse the Y Corridor would muster all strength, largely from support and encouragement of leaving family members, to complete the journey ahead alongside steadfast medical personnel.

As immigration increased at Ellis Island, medical advancements abounded and resources to advance the cause improved. The call for another hospital to be built on site emerged. With the final expansions for the hospital located on Island 2 completed, the only direction for expansion was the southern view from atop the Spanish terracotta-lined porticos. Soon enough, across from this view, a wide man-made lagoon would be built to the new Island 3.

Much like the original small strip of land connecting the immigration center on Island 1 to the General Health Hospital on Island 2, a similar section of land would be laid out to connect Island 2 to the new Island 3. Island 3 would become the future home for the newly constructed Contagious and Infectious Disease Hospital at Ellis Island.

Before patients were ever admitted to the

Contagious Disease Hospital, their journey at Ellis Island would begin in the immigration center on Island 1.

Members of the Public Health Service stationed in the immigration center served at the frontline, utilizing their gaze through the Great Hall for those who may pose a threat to public health. The finest medical instrument at their disposal would be the staircase through which immigrants made their way up to the second floor. They would station themselves at every turn of the staircase to observe which immigrants struggled to make the climb. Using the natural lighting in the open stairwell as it directly hit the faces of the immigrants at each turn, doctors would be able to see if they appeared grey and haggard or were suffering jaundice. This group of people, along with those exhibiting heavy steps up the winding stairs and gasping for breath, would unfortunately see the end of their heroic voyage.

These doctors in military uniform were not holding rifles or swords but a steady piece of white chalk at their side. With a quick assessment done by the Public Health Service as they rounded the stairs, doctors would mark the lapel or the back of the immigrant with their medical opinion in short order. An immigrant exhibiting signs of a limp as he made the climb would be marked as 'L' for lameness while an immigrant hunched over or in pain would be marked as 'B' for back. Both would be sent for further examination but both would be at risk for deportation due to apprehension of being a public charge.

The Public Health Service would break these two types of markings that would be chalked onto an immigrant into two distinct categories. The "'Class A' [being the] loathsome or dangerous contagious diseases and 'Class B' diseases being conditions that would render an immigrant likely to become a public charge."[32] With plans for a Contagious Disease Hospital underway and the goal to be completed in the peak year of 1907, these two categories could now be separated further.

The plan would call for the construction of the additional soil gangplank to be built no less than 200 feet from the General Health Hospital on Island 2 southwards. With this distance, it was believed, under the thinking of the time by the very best medical experts, that this would be sufficient distance over clear water to not allow any transference of contagious diseases. From here, an island of similar stature and size would be built for Island 3 at Ellis Island and would be the new home for the Contagious Disease Hospital to treat patients from far and wide.

For the patients who would soon call this place home, they would be marked with the Class A chalk marks. With a Public Health Service doctor seeing blood on the shirt sleeve of an immigrant or hearing a wheezing cough as they made their way up the stairs to the Great Hall, they would be quickly marked with a 'P' on their back for 'Physical and Lungs' to be examined for a potentially fatal disease of the time.

A patient diagnosed with the likes of tuberculosis would perhaps be saying goodbye to their family for the very last time as they made their way to the hospital complex at Ellis Island. It was likely for that patient to be sent back home as there was no known cure for tuberculosis and the patient's inability to pay for prolonged treatment. As Class A diseases were not treated for free, a long stay for treatment of tuberculosis, also known as consumption, could be far too much for a family who had risked it all on the American dream to pay. The immigration service believed that since it was the responsibility of the shipping company to run a clean and hygienic business, it was also the shipping company's responsibility to take the severely-sick person back home. The return would often be in far harsher conditions than when they first traveled to the United States. Worse, these immigrants would have no families or properties to return to. Aside from transporting them back home, a fine of $200 per person admitted with a loathsome disease (in 1900) was imposed upon the responsible shipping company.

For the shipping companies to avoid the looming threat of a monetary fine and figuring out ways to avoid transporting an individual with a contagious disease, they often had doctors in their employ board the ship at the point of departure. These physicians, who were known to be far less friendly and kind than those found at Ellis Island, would intimidate any boarding immigrants who knew that they could be suffering from any infectious disease. The hope was to detour these immigrants who thought they could stake their hopes on the fresh air of the new world to cure them of their ailment. Shipping companies would also strive to make the journey to America safer by designating decks for fresh air based on class and employing extermination crews to fight off seafaring rats who were known to carry foul diseases.

For those who would still catch one of these diseases and would not be cleared by the Public Health Service to leave the Island, they were directed towards Island 2 where they would be greeted by the infamous Y Corridor. This fork in the road was designed to separate Class A from Class B diseases for the very first time at Ellis Island. The turn to the left would lead to the General Health Hospital where health issues, not as grave as to render a patient a public charge, would be treated. The turn to the right would lead to a journey across the soil gangplank and a 200 foot long walk up into the Contagious Disease Hospital on Island 3.

With landfill, rocks, and soil still in plenty

from construction projects in New York City, the Island 3 hospital complex would be built out much the same way as Island 2. The first structure planned was to build a central admitting building and dormitory space right in the middle of Island 3. The structure would be constructed using concrete and steel - a much more utilitarian fashion to last the test of time. This new construction showed the advancements happening across the country and the ability to quickly construct strong buildings. With a concrete pebble exterior and large windows, this hospital would have an opposing look for immigrants as they drew closer to the Island through the harbor.

A total of sixteen wards would be built around the completed central admitting building. To transport patients from the central admitting to the wards, a 'hand-ambulance' would be devised which included a 'prairie schooner top' covering the patient who would be warm under sterile blankets. This design would keep them from spreading or picking up any germs on the way to the wards.

The wards would be constructed in a staggered fashion so they would never be directly across from one another. This design was to avoid a draft spreading disease across the hall. To connect them to one another, they would lead out onto a central corridor that united them all to the 'spine' of the hospital. Within the wards, they would follow a similar fashion to using an open ward design common of the early 20th century. With twelve, fourteen, and sometimes sixteen patient beds wrapped around the room, the space would still feel spacious with the tall windows and ceilings. The wards would measure 55 feet long by 27 feet wide to provide adequate spacing for patients. As detailed in the book *The Modern Hospital,* spacing would allow for "45 square feet of floor space for each child 3 to 4 years of age, 65 square feet for children over 4, and 80 square feet for adults. The height of the walls [would be] sufficient to give a cubic air space of over 1,000 feet per adult and a correspondingly liberal amount for children."[33] This ward design would remain the same except for those dedicated for the treatment of tuberculosis which would use already established single patient rooms.

The single patient wards using partitions would quickly become the norm and would not only give patients isolation and privacy, but would give nurses the ability to oversee more patients. J.G Wilson, a doctor with the Public Health Service at Ellis Island, noted that the large open wards would often prove ineffective in treating contagious diseases. "Although opened to receive patients in June, 1911, the [Contagious Disease] hospital [was] still in the process of making, large wards being divided into smaller, and interior alterations being made in order to evolve gradually a more perfect system of isolation units."[33] Overtime, partitions would be constructed to provide separation among patients. To that end, they would also use some of the previously constructed nurses' quarters which were also single-capacity rooms.

Wards in the hospital would be designated by their disease as outbreaks would come and go. They would be split up into dedicated spaces for measles, scarlet fever, and whooping cough, and further broken out by gender. Within the two-story wards, females and those under the age of twelve would be housed on one floor, and men would be housed on the other. The wards would all follow a strict concept of patient distancing, fresh air, and natural sunlight through the large open windows. The Contagious Disease Hospital at Ellis Island, once complete, would house five hundred patient beds - massive even for hospitals today in America.

For those with far more contagious diseases, the stay was often much more isolating and lonely. For young children fighting a scalp disease called favus, an eye infection called trachoma, or tuberculosis, the stay was often far less pleasant compounded with great fear of being sent back.

As the patients were escorted through the long concrete corridor, stretching a sprawling 800 feet, the journey to the far end to isolation would be a scary walk. Prior to the Contagious Disease Hospital being fully complete in 1911, there would be no glass installed in the windows throughout its wide two-story hallway. Thus, the walk could even involve watching for patches of snow and ice. To get to the isolation ward with single patient housing, one would walk through the hall, passing the steel doors of measles wards while smelling the roasting of vegetables from the single kitchen and hearing laughter from the nurse's quarters.

Upon entering any of the wards, the layout would be very much the same. Nurse's offices, small dispensary, restrooms, and a shower room would lead into a large open and cavernous room in a standard ward. But the isolation wards were quite different. As opposed to the open ward, these were designed as single patient quarters. With a steel door that could be locked from the internal hall, patients would scarcely have room for much more than a bed. Patients admitted to the tuberculosis wards would be surprised to find two sinks in their room. Many of these patients barely lived in a home with any sink at all prior to their journey to America. What was even more peculiar was that one of the two sinks would be higher on the wall and slightly smaller than the other. This top sink would serve a more unpleasant purpose, that is, to cough and spit blood and sputum into. Lined with rags to be burnt in the incinerator or let to drain, this would bring a putrid smell to an already sad room.

Treatment options would vary for these poor souls even with advances in science occurring. "On March 24, 1882, Dr. Robert Koch announced the discovery of *Mycobacterium tuberculosis*, the bacteria that causes tuberculosis (TB). During this time, TB killed one out of every seven people living in the United States and Europe."[34] This dreadful disease had been around for millennia with varied attempts at treatment but no known cure.

Treatment options would come in the form of sanatoriums. These centers would crop up where they could offer relief from the pain and fatigue brought on by this debilitating disease. Often located in beautiful and airy mountain retreats, these sanatoriums would often be out of reach for poor immigrants barely able to afford housing. Fresh air and sunlight would be the kindest options to offer relief. Many institutions would rely on much more rudimentary treatments such as inhaling medicinal concoctions or, worse, collapsing a lung to allow it to rest.

With little to no options, these poor immigrants would become outcasts and with more public education, persecution against them would rise. The crowded cities would do much to teach of sanitation and clean air to ward off the vile disease. It would not be until 1943, with the advent of antibiotics, that physicians would finally have a weapon to fight back with a cure.

Another such troublesome disease would be that of favus which would impact children suffering itching of a fungus on their scalps. In the immigrant hospitals, further isolation wards down the hall would offer them care. Favus, a fungal disease presenting often on the scalp in the form of a rough honeycomb shaped patch, would prove to be a great challenge. This was a common issue for those who were not used to bathing on a regular basis and the long voyage at sea would not help. As favus was more of a chronic disease that, in some cases, would take years to treat and cure, it was often a ground for deportation for the youngest of immigrants.

However, if treatment was attempted, it was not always pleasant for the patient. Measures would call for experimental treatment of using x-rays to repeatedly blast the head with radiation to burn the fungal disease. Other options would be to remove the hair follicles where the fungus was located. A topical treatment to help recover from these harsh options would be the application of a pitch cap. The cap was made from a solution of tree sap which was not often easy to remove once applied.

Worse than favus would be the loathsome disease of trachoma. The buttonhook, which was normally used for fastening of shoes, would be repurposed to examine for this disease, making this new 'medical' instrument famously intertwined with the history of Ellis Island.

Trachoma was one of the most unique and troublesome infectious diseases to be seen at Ellis Island given how it was examined. To check if an immigrant had it, Public Health Service doctors would invert the eyelids of the immigrant looking for the telltale signs of red eyes, scaring under the eyelid and, in some cases, a discharge of pus. To note, despite the infectious nature of trachoma, the need to disinfect the buttonhook used to examine it was not immediately obvious to the doctors.

Before immigrants would disembark at Ellis Island, trachoma would have already spread like wildfire in route. This is because these immigrants would use the same towels, bedding, and would be in close contact with each other. With repeated infection, the eyelashes would literally turn inside out, scraping the person's eye with each and every blink in the dazzling sun at sea. Overtime, this would lead to a painful and eventual blindness which would mean difficulty finding work in the early 1900's. In America, this would be equal to being called a public charge and being sent home.

Treatments of trachoma had not evolved much over the course of history prior to and even during the time of Ellis Island. In fact, today, it is still common in Latin America, Africa, the Middle East and Asia. Back then, doctors would use what was called the 'blue stone,' which was copper sulfate in a crystalline form mounted to a small brush handle. By inverting the eyelid and repeatedly scouring the tissue with this course stone, remission was sometimes possible. However, it would take months to treat and would often require recurring treatments. Thankfully today, if detected early, trachoma could be cured through antibiotics.

However, not all diseases at Ellis Island would be as painful as tuberculosis, favus, and trachoma. For some, the care they received was truly memorable. Many children who were lonely, scared, and afraid in the hospital would be nurtured and loved by nurses. For many nurses, the practice of kissing a child's forehead to determine fever was commonplace, but could be a deadly practice in any contagious disease hospital. Rules would be implemented to encourage nurses not to practice this technique and to avoid hugging patients, not because of indifference but out of precaution to ensure their health and safety. Nurses were also encouraged to not do things which may seem trivial at that time such as sharing pencils or instruments used in other wards so as to avoid spreading disease.

Many techniques were being implemented to avoid cross contamination and the spread of disease at Ellis Island. Florence Nightingale deserves much of the credit for her modernization in nursing and focus on sanitation.

Nightingale was a nurse who would rise to prominence in the mid-19th century for her work during the Crimean War in Europe. At that time, she would hear screaming not from the battle waging but from patients battling infections from earlier battle wounds. She would witness patients' sufferings exacerbated by how they were cared for in seldom more than squalor circumstances. "She became known as the 'Lady with the Lamp' because of her night rounds. While nursing soldiers during the war, Nightingale worked to improve nutrition and conditions in the wards."[35] The time was quickly becoming ripe for hospitals to become a place of hope and not of pain and loss.

With advancements in sterilization occurring, the long corridor connecting the wards together down the spine of the hospital would be a first line of defense for patients and staff. With the hurried pace of a nurse, her white shoes clicking against the smooth concrete would echo down the pathway in the summer breeze.

Standing at one end, the 800-foot corridor would present an amazing and opposing view for a new patient or staff. Looking towards the horizon, it would appear smaller which made perfect sense. However, the hall would actually in fact get smaller going from west to east. This was a stroke of brilliance as it was designed to create a good flow of air, forming a ventilation chamber by opening windows and doors at either end. By keeping this steady flow of air, disease and germs could be easily dispelled out. Surrounded by the concrete hall, the drains in the floors would also allow for easy mopping and sterilization of the walls and floors on a daily basis.

The same halls would serve as the path for

carts to be rolled busily with healthy meals from the central kitchen in the hospital. With the kitchen on Island 3 situated right against the southern edge of the Island, supply boats would be able to bring in fresh produce and dairy from the 'Garden State' of New Jersey close by. With the milk and fresh vegetables being the staple for busy New Yorkers, this would prove to be a vital nutrient to immigrants who were fighting scurvy from poor diets while in route to America. Thus, many of them would be seeing new tropical fruits like bananas for the very first time in an effort to achieve a balanced diet. There were tales of immigrants who would either bite straight through the skin of a banana or who would think of spaghetti as a plate of worms upon their first encounter with these new foods. Thankfully, Ettore Boiardi, who would later become the famous 'Chef Boyardee,' would come through Ellis Island in 1914 to educate future generations about Italian meals.

Orderlies would move large carts of food from the kitchen to each ward where nurses and staff would be able to plate up healthy and nutritious meals for weary patients. However, each ward would have its own set of plates and utensils that would be used and washed in that area alone. In that way, only the empty serving trays would go back, avoiding anything with patient germs to contaminate the central kitchen utensils and space.

In addition to the central kitchen for each

hospital, a kosher kitchen would be housed on Island 1 near the bakery. The kitchen would serve kosher meals to Jewish immigrants.

Aside from a systematic meal production, the hospital would also be equipped with facilities to help patients get excellent rest. Patients' beds would be placed between wide open windows to allow light to flood in. Below each window would be a large steam radiator to warm the cold air coming in. This would prove to be a good remedy for those with weakened bodies from their cold and drafty voyage.

The hospital also took sanitation seriously per Florence Nightingale's teachings. With medicines from the dispensary onsite still being rudimentary, using clean beds for rest would often reap the greatest benefits. To ensure a clean and sterile place to rest, the Island would operate a mattress autoclave to steam clean the mattresses. Used mattresses would be placed inside the vault-like machine and staff would spin the wheels to securely lock the doors. With the autoclave being right next to the power plant on the Island, it would be able to blast the mattresses with high pressure steam to sterilize and kill germs from the previous patient. Mattresses would then be put on hooks to hang to be air-dried.

People then recognized that a clean mattress was nothing without crisp clean sheets. Thus, the laundry facilities on Island 2 would be a busy place with staff cleaning, pressing, and folding over two thousand pieces of bedding and clothing a day at a very efficient rate of $.01 per piece. With the laundry facility putting out pressed sheets, nurses could combat the ever growing concern of bedsores on patients lying on dirty or loose fitting bed sheets. This could have been a death sentence prior to the days of antibiotics for immigrant patients.

Surgeon General medical records and other historical accounts would show the great lengths that medical staff went to serve patients at Ellis Island. In numerous journal entries and recorded testimonies, former patients would often refer to nurses as 'angels' on the Island. With doctors and nurses living on site, their shifts never seemed to end and, for many, helping those less fortunate would become more of a calling.

Despite the extraordinary work of the doctors at Ellis Island, some patients would not be so fortunate. Records kept by the Public Health Service note 5,435 deaths in the hospitals. Any death was of course tragic, but it is remarkable that this figure was out of a total of over 416,000 patients that were admitted to the hospitals at Ellis Island. This would equate to a mortality rate of 1.3 percent of patients! While this rate is impressive, one needs to recall that the shipping companies carrying the immigrants to America employed doctors to screen immigrants as they boarded the vessel. Thus, the sickest of the sick would have never made the journey in the first place and this probably contributed to the low mortality rate at Ellis Island.

To handle the dead, a large autopsy amphitheater would be constructed at the southwestern edge of the Contagious Disease Hospital (right below the doctors' quarters). On the back wall of the autopsy room, coat hooks would run the full length for physicians to hang their lab coats after a day's work.

Interestingly, the autopsy room would also serve as a 'classroom.' At the center of the room would be a table with a gas light above. Behind it would be eight coolers used to preserve dead bodies and in front of it would be three tiers of wooden seating where doctors would observe from above. From the eight coolers, doctors would retrieve a dead body for examination to understand new diseases and their impacts. The autopsy room would be painted in dark green on the lower half and white on the upper half. This green paint would allow for any blood splatter to be quickly seen and cleaned. The white paint against the large windows going across the western wall would allow the setting sun to draw long shadows of light across the room.

Once the autopsy examination was completed, the body would be wrapped in sheets coated in antiseptic to be removed from the Island. If families could afford proper burial it would be offered, but often, with limited resources, many immigrants would find their final resting place at Hart Island. This island would serve as a potter's field located at the northern tip of the city on the East River.

As the 1920's approached, additional landfill would be barged over to Ellis Island to fill in the lagoon that previously created a barrier for disease between Islands 2 and 3. This would provide patients spacious grounds to get more exercise and fresh air. Tales would be told of beautiful gardens between the gravel walks and the Daughters of the American Revolution sponsoring a sack race for patients. The expanded lawn would also allow for a tennis court to be constructed for the doctors.

As the grounds would be open to both patients and staff, the co-habitation would allow for deeper bonds to be developed, lightening the impact of the immigrants' separation from family and friends. In addition to the recreation centers during the Great Depression, an outdoor pavilion would be constructed for patients to take in the refreshing and peaceful outdoor air - thanks to the WPA (Works Progress Administration). The handsome brick terrace would allow for patients to take in the harbor views from the shade. To add to this, just to the west of it, an ornate indoor facility fitted with a stage and projection booth would be constructed. Ellis Island would advertise the safety of the hospitals to entice Broadway actors and actresses to come in and perform for patients.

During World War I, immigration would nearly come to a halt with the passing of the 1917 Immigration Act. Congress would enact one of the first broadly restrictive immigration laws since the late 19th century. "This law is best known for its creation of a 'barred zone' extending from the Middle East to Southeast Asia from which no persons were allowed to enter the United States. Its main restriction, however, consisted of a literacy test intended to reduce European immigration, with exemptions for those who could show they were fleeing persecution."[36] With fears of radicalism in Europe and a world at war, immigration would be nearly shut off.

Activities on the Island would begin to quickly transition from being focused on immigration to being more oriented towards medical care for merchant marines. "In September 1919 the U. S. Public Health Service assumed control of the hospital from the Department of Labor and operated it as marine 'Hospital No. 43.' The transfer agreement stipulated that immigrant patients would continue to have precedence in admission over other patients, including U. S. seamen, although by 1929 most patients were affiliated with the Merchant Marine or U. S. Coast Guard and only twenty-five percent of the patients were immigrants."[37]

As the hospitals were originally constructed via the Marine Hospital Fund, the evolution of the Island was actually natural. For the first time, Ellis Island would now begin to see more patients from military backgrounds and fewer immigrants. It would start to see a change of the guard in its use. However, the hospitals' main purpose of treating all those who entered its doors with dignity and respect was only growing stronger.

Despite all the changes at that time, the Island would not be silenced and would remain relevant. It would assist in training nurses prior to disembarking for a tour in the war in Europe. For those returning from war, the hospitals would serve as a place of recovery. It would even see the addition of an occupational therapy ward as early as 1917. This would be right around the very first meeting of the National Society for the Promotion of Occupational Therapy (NSPOT) at Clifton Springs in upstate New York. With pianos and looms, doctors could work with patients dealing with war fatigue and help them find peace from the battlefield.

The greatest decline in immigration would only be a few years removed from World War I. The Immigration Act of 1924 would further limit the number of immigrants allowed entry into the United States. Pursuant to the Act, a national origins quota was implemented. Specifically, the quota limited the issuance of immigration visas to only two percent of each nationality who were in the United States as of the 1890 national census. This measure caused a significant drop in the number of immigrants previously flooding through Ellis Island.

As the Great War had proven, no one was out of reach of a war of indifference. As America had demonstrated its ability to be a global power during World War I, the 1924 Act would seek to make sure wages stayed high for citizens by cutting off the immigrants from the labor pool. This was the political view of the then administration to ensure that the roaring 20's could roar on…until they came to a screeching halt in 1929.

As the Great Depression took hold, America would no longer be the land of opportunity it had once been as there would simply be no opportunity to even be had. Some would still try and make the journey. The global economy would be brought to its knees and some world leaders would point blame on the Jews for the demise of businesses and industries. This persecution would bring refugees to America as the country would still be viewed then as the last best hope of the world.

Ellis Island would never see again huddled masses of immigrants seeking a better life nor would the hospital wards be filled with languages and dialects from around the world. The peak years of immigration at Ellis Island would simply run from 1900 to 1914 and would only ever grow to 33 buildings dotting the Island landscape. This Island and its historic buildings still stand as a tribute today for future generations to marvel at how the story of their ancestors began in America. The stories of the immigrants who once passed through the doors of Ellis Island are a testament to their great sacrifices.

PART III: THE END OF AN ERA OF ELLIS ISLAND IMMIGRATION

CHAPTER 7: THE END OF ELLIS IMMIGRATION

> "Your grandparents came of age in the Great Depression, when everyday life was about deprivation and sacrifice, when the economic conditions of the time were so grave and so unrelenting it would have been easy enough for the American dream to fade away."
>
> -Tom Brokaw

The American dream was beginning to look more and more like a dream unobtainable – even for those already in America. This early 1930's was beginning to become the era of thriving big businesses and immigrants at that time were viewed only by the 'value' they brought to an enterprise. The perspective that an immigrant was only important to the bottom line was not new at all. However, it was exacerbated during the growth of the Industrial Revolution. From the depths of the Panama Canal, railroads crisscrossing the west, to skyscrapers now touching the sky, immigrants would be the first ones in to do the heavy work.

However, with stricter and stricter regulations on who could get into the country, there would only be a trickle of immigrants seeking refuge in America. These new immigrants would still make their way in through Ellis Island as they would not be able to go through a consulate in their country of origin. The hospitals would begin to only see the sickest immigrant patients suffering from tuberculosis coupled with psychiatric health concerns. Having such a weakened mental state would not be uncommon for patients suffering a debilitating disease such as tuberculosis.

"As a result of the Great Depression, minorities were [being] blamed for the economic downturn and began to be targeted for layoffs as well as deportations and hate crimes. This blaming was placed on Chinese, Japanese, and Mexican immigrants, as well as other immigrants throughout the 1930s."[38]

This was not to say that the challenge faced by non-immigrants was any lighter. One race in particular, the African Americans, who already had limited rights saw even tougher challenges during the depression. While no group would be able to escape the economic devastation of the Great

Depression, no one would endure it harder than the African Americans. "Said to be 'last hired, first fired,' African Americans were the first to see hours and jobs cut, and they experienced the highest unemployment rate during the 1930s."[39]

It has long been determined that shuttering a nation's doors during decline and placing restrictions on commerce and movement would be more of a hindrance than a help to economic recovery. Restricting immigration, along with the ideas that come from this easy movement, could cause a country in isolation, economic challenges and a drop in free enterprise.

As immigration at all ports declined, the facilities at Ellis Island would begin to see less and less traffic. It would not be until the approach of World War II when immigration would begin to pick back up to a peak of just over sixty thousand immigrants a year seeking refuge from religious persecution in Europe.

Through war raging abroad, Ellis Island would become eerily silent as everyone's focus turned to the battles overseas. During this time, it would see its greatest use as a Coast Guard training center. Service members would use the Great Hall of the immigration center to rest on bunks installed before shipping out. The hospitals would begin to see ivy climb the limestone and weeds sprouting amongst the early gardens. Rust would begin to eat away the screens installed on windows and at the playground space for children.

As the war was ending and peace talks were beginning, the chance for Ellis Island to be used again as an immigration center was reemerging. However, immigration, as well as the medicines used to treat loathsome diseases, were both quickly modernizing in this new peacetime era. It would be a cold November day in 1954, that the last person to depart the hospitals would be a Norwegian merchant seaman. The former Contagious Disease Hospital wards would be used in a limited capacity with even an indoor basketball court being installed in one of the upper floor wards. It would go from a center of welcome to one of farewell. Numerous pieces of legislation would cause Ellis Island to change from a processing center for immigrants to a detention and deportation facility for illegal immigrants.

The Island would be shuttered as the United States government would begin to take stock of surplus properties which unfortunately included Ellis Island for potential sale. With the nation growing more rapidly, resources would be needed to keep up with funding the new interstate program allowing for easier movement. This Island, where so much history was made, was seen as no longer of significance in this new time.

Now that Ellis Island was abandoned, the opportunity was left to the highest bidder and developer for the site. One such offer was presented and even plans drawn up by the famous architect, Frank Lloyd Wright. He would present plans for a modern city, with towering hotels, apartments, and parks that would have truly changed the landscape of the Island had the offer been accepted.

However, none of the plans would be deemed suitable. It would be in 1963 that a proposal would be made by New York City Mayor Robert F. Wagner to preserve this site as a historical landmark. It would take until 1964 for the Department of Interior to approve the National Parks Service proposal to add this site as part of the Statue of Liberty National Monument.

Initially, only limited funds would be set aside to conduct emergency repairs to an already crumbling island. The salt water air was taking its toll on the old buildings which had seen hard use. With no real direction on repairing or restoring the site, Ellis Island would only see limited visitation of the crumbling memorial. As it was only a short quarter mile from the shores of New Jersey, stories of those who would row out to the island to look around were not uncommon.

It would not be until May of 1982 that President Ronald Reagan would announce plans for the formation of the Statue of Liberty – Ellis Island Centennial Commission to restore these national treasures. With Lee Iacocca taking charge, fundraising would begin for the much needed restoration. Plans called for the renovations of the main immigration processing center and creating a museum that would tell the story of immigration for future generations.

After years of fundraising and sourcing skilled craftsman, on September 10, 1990, the main immigration center would be returned to its former glory. For the first time, families could walk in the steps of their ancestors through the echoing halls of Ellis Island. As they typed in computers terminals, they could see the historic manifest appear on their screen showing their family's entry into America. As visitors to the National Park would hear from ranger-led tours, it would not be on the Island that the names of immigrants would be changed, but perhaps in the home country as they departed. They would also learn that there was no big book of signatures like in the movies as Hollywood just created these fables. Work would continue to be ongoing to restore the ferry building and other historic spaces at Ellis Island.

As guests awaited their next ferry after a day of learning their ancestry, they could not help but ponder the history of the buildings on the south side of Ellis Island.

Funds would not be sufficient to restore the south side of Ellis Island and this would be deemed a restricted zone for guests to the National Park. It would require the likes of a non-profit, Save Ellis Island, to make plans to bring about restoration and rehabilitation. The organization's plan would at the very least try to arrest the decay from spreading. They would endeavor to become a park partner, hosting hard hat tours of the immigrant hospitals in an effort to raise funds and tell the stories of these forgotten buildings.

The very latest accomplishment came in 2019 when the Recreation Building, which was originally built by the WPA between 1933 and 1937, had been fully renovated. This pavilion was built on top of what was the original lagoon between the islands originally used by patients to find cover on sunny days. Today, hopefully, it is now a stop for tours for the next generation. Through the famous hard hat tours and grants, the organization of Save Ellis Island continues to seek ways to preserve this side of the Island before it is too late.

This quest has become even more important in recent years. In October of 2012, the entire Island would be flooded in up to waist deep water from the super storm, Hurricane Sandy. With rains and winds tearing at the Spanish terracotta roofs of the immigrant hospitals, windowpanes were pelted to the point of breaking and the damage would nearly condemn these amazing pieces of history.

As each winter passes, the freezing and thawing spring brings more decay to the beautiful buildings.

The original skylights that would have allowed light to flood into the top floor operating rooms have long since been broken away and now rains are able to flood in. The warm summer breezes full of salty air bring more and more rust to the old iron and uncertainty of the future of the hospitals. The need for hard hats on tours of the buildings becomes more and more of a necessity and less of a fashion statement.

As there continues to be a risk of rising ocean waters, this Island remains in jeopardy from the next super-storm. To preserve Ellis Island for the next generation, it is vital that efforts remain underway to repair and restore the seawall protecting the buildings. It is only by knowing the history and importance of Ellis Island can we begin to understand what the world would have looked like had it actually slipped below the waters of the Hudson before it even had begun to be a mecca for many wanting to know their family's story.

Today, the halls still echo with the languages of afar. Schoolchildren bound through the exhibits and see displays of now antique baggage, letters, and tools of the era of Ellis Island Immigration. Videos show the processing of immigrants from a century ago and recorded oral histories can be found in the Bob Hope Library. If you are lucky enough to take a ranger tour, you may get to jokingly hear how Annie Moore pushed Ranger Sam out of the way from being the first immigrant to make it through processing over a century ago.

The history and lessons from the sacrifices made by many immigrants who went through this site shall never be forgotten.

CHAPTER 8: ISLAND OF HOPE - FORGOTTEN

> "Our attitude towards immigration reflects our faith in the American ideal. We have always believed it possible for men and women who start at the bottom to rise as far as the talent and energy allow. Neither race nor place of birth should affect their chances."
> - Robert F. Kennedy

As I walk the halls of the Ellis Island Contagious Disease Hospital on a cool autumn afternoon, a modern-day doctor participates in my tour. My tour today is presented to the New York College of Medicine. As we are about to enter a tuberculosis ward, with our hard hats glinting in the setting sun, he tells a tale I would recount on nearly every tour to follow. In a humble voice, he tells his students that when he was in medical school, he studied treatments for tuberculosis. His son would follow in his footsteps and pursued the same profession. He tells that when his son was in medical school, the pursuit was to find treatment for AIDS. Beaming with pride, he mentions that his grandson, who is next in line, will be exploring the treatment for cancer. As a smile crept over his face, he exclaimed how one could not be optimistic knowing that tale! Indeed, it is remarkable how each and every generation of physicians gets to face a new disease, a new challenge. To them, it is perhaps a great blessing that God has a purpose for their time.

I would go on to recount this story to each and every one of my succeeding tours. I would of course preface it by saying that this story was from the second favorite tour I ever had the privilege of giving – second only to the one I was presently giving!

The doctors at Ellis Island were on the cutting edge of their profession and their dedication to humanity was second to none. Without them, the immigrants who came would not have the same chance of success. Even if Ellis Island may go by the nickname of the 'Island of Hope, Island of Tears,' to me, it was more of a hopeful island which prepared immigrants to only have tears of joy by the new opportunities that awaited them. By providing a process for transition, rather than dropping immigrants right in the middle of New York City, Ellis Island truly set them up for success and better lives.

As immigrants finished processing on the Island, they would have the option to visit a ticketing office on the Island to purchase train tickets for the next leg of their journey. Whether going into the hustle and bustle of New York City or going to the shores of New Jersey to travel west, these offices would provide help to get these immigrants to where opportunity existed. The site would also offer amenities such as a small café where immigrants could have a hot meal at a decent cost, a money exchange, and even numerous support services run by aid societies.

The aid societies at Ellis Island offered guidance, food, clothing, and religious services to immigrants coming to this new land. "Organizations assisting immigrants on the Island included the *Young Women's Christian Association* (YWCA), the *Young Men's Christian Association* (YMCA), the *Daughters of the American Revolution* (DAR), *the Salvation Army*, and the *Traveler's Aid Society*. Additionally there were culturally specific needs met by ethnic Italian, German, Polish, Lithuanian and Spanish branches of the Roman Catholic Church's *St. Raphael's Society*, the *Hebrew Immigrant Aid Society* (HIAS) and National Council of Jewish Women, the *White Rose Mission*, specifically for Caribbean women, and various other societies exclusively for Belgians, Bulgarians, Dutch, Greeks, Italians, Hungarians, Poles and Russians."[40]

These aid societies would offer much advice in which way to go, one which may serve the immigrant best. A story goes that an older hunched-over immigrant said he planned to go to Pennsylvania to make his fortune in the growing coal mines. When speaking with an aid worker, they promptly gave him advice that perhaps he would be of better service to his family as a tailor in the expanding garment district. These simple discussions saved countless lives and set many families to truly experience the American dream.

For immigrants leaving Ellis Island via another quick ferry ride, they could find themselves at the Central Railroad of New Jersey Terminal. This terminal, like many others going up the waterfront, would allow immigrants the option to travel west across the growing country if they did not wish to settle in the big cities. Today, visitors to Ellis Island and the Statue of Liberty can still see the remains of this historic terminal in Liberty State Park. A few miles up the river, the Hoboken Terminal, which was opened precisely during the peak year of immigration at Ellis Island in 1907, is still in use today.

Even with the chance to go west, many immigrants would plan to stake their claim in the big cities. To these people who would look to make the urban centers their home, the reality of sickness and squalor in tenement housing and other urban challenges would not stop them from seeking the opportunities that were available there.

Despite the growing abuses of capitalism, immigrants would not be quick to voice their issues, believing deep in their hearts that it was through hard work that they could offer their families better lives.

However, as time passed, immigrants would band together - with language and religion as a common core - to push for equal rights and equal pay. Through bloody strikes, factory fires, working in deep dark mines and towering on steel beams reaching to the sun, these immigrants risked their lives to prove the American dream was worth chasing. Their sweat, tears, and blood would make these cities what they have become today – a slightly fairer place to do business. Indeed, the sacrifices of these immigrants should not be forgotten.

However, no matter how great the challenges the immigrants faced in America, they were able to find comfort in bringing with them memories of home. Whether from the likes of Alphabet City, Chinatown, or Little Italy in lower Manhattan, Italian, German-baked goods, and countless other cuisines would provide comforts from home. These same neighborhoods still provide these delicacies today where they still reign supreme.

The cities across America today still embrace the legacy that these immigrants brought in the form of making America a melting pot. Unique cultures, ideas and imaginings were brought together over a hot meal at the end of a long day. Within New York City alone, a 2010 New York Times article notes that "some experts believe New York is home to as many as 800 languages - far more than the 176 spoken by students in the city's public schools or the 138 that residents of Queens, New York's most diverse borough, listed on their 2000 census forms."[41]

Through all the things that Ellis Island offered, may it be in the form of medical care, assistance, or a threshold to this new land, this island of hope was able to give immigrants a fighting chance. It was truly a promising place that changed the world we live in today and makes America, as Abraham Lincoln once said, "the last best hope of the earth."

CHAPTER 9: WHY IT MATTERS TODAY

> "The bosom of America is open to receive not only the Opulent and respected Stranger, but the oppressed and persecuted of all Nations and Religions; whom we shall welcome to a participation of all our rights and privileges..."
> – President George Washington

So, what would the likes of New York City or Hoboken, New Jersey look like today had Ellis Island simply washed away and never become more than a small rocky island in the harbor?

To understand what life would have been like without Ellis Island, we must recall what it was like in the years before it even opened. One can say that as early as the dawn of the nation, New York City was already a 'city that never slept' because of all the taverns and unsavory activities happening in every corner. In fact, as General George Washington would set up his encampments at lower Manhattan to defend New York City in 1776, his greatest challenge, aside from facing a much more able enemy, was to keep his ragtag army healthy and focused in this recalcitrant city.

Prior to Ellis Island, there was also a very limited immigration process. Much of the reason that Ellis Island's predecessor, the original Castle Garden, shuttered was its lack of a structured and holistic approach to welcoming (or rejecting) immigrants. An immigrant who arrived at the port sick, or who was a passenger onboard a vessel that had a disease outbreak, would not have easy access to treatment; instead, he likely would be trapped onboard a 'Death Ship' laying at anchor in the harbor. An immigrant who was otherwise admitted upon arrival was very much left to figure out on his own how to find accommodation and work once he walked out of Castle Garden.

It is also very important to highlight that during the years preceding Ellis Island, disease was very rampant in New York City. At that time, New York's Bellevue Hospital would strive to address the issue. The hospital would attempt to introduce cutting-edge innovations in medical science, particularly in the fight against contagious diseases. It would build amphitheaters, medical college and a nursing school. In 1869, the Bellevue Hospital would implement the first ambulatory service in the nation -- a horse drawn ambulance ready to trot into action. Per their commission, "each ambulance shall have a box beneath the driver's seat, containing a quart flask of brandy, two tourniquets, a half-dozen bandages, a half-dozen small sponges, some splint material, pieces of old blankets for padding, strips of various lengths with buckles, and a two-ounce vial of persulphate of iron."[42] Despite these developments, Bellevue Hospital, with limited resources, only went so far in preventing outbreak and the spread of contagious diseases in New York City.

It is against this background that I would like to imagine what it would have looked like for an immigrant coming to America if Ellis Island was never built. Let us explore this scenario.

Without Ellis Island, an immigrant would walk through and out of Castle Garden. As he was not provided with a currency exchange facility (which Ellis Island did), he would look to have his money exchanged with the first respectable-looking person to approach him. The immigrant would probably be short-changed but he would have no choice; he would need a meal before looking for housing a short distance from the dark and grimy factories that may exist in the city. Unarmed with any advice or help from aid organizations that Ellis Island provided, the immigrant would have no guide in understanding work opportunities or would have no clue to even understand what awaits him in the city aside from a basic pamphlet.

Walking away from the river's edge, the

immigrant would approach the nearest street market crowded with wooden carts. Scanning the market, he would be curious to see what appeared to be fresh fruits, vegetables, and meat on display for sale. However, upon closer examination, he would see the circling of houseflies over brown rotten-meat and sour spoiled-milk. Without having the benefit of getting rest post voyage or receiving appropriate treatment if he was feeling unwell from an Ellis Island facility, the health of this tired and weak immigrant would probably just deteriorate. With gutters lined with sewage from both animal and human, the summer heat would make the air unpleasant to breath. However, with dreams of a soft warm bed in a tenement house, the immigrant would probably power through and weave his way through the crowded streets filled with filth. The immigrant would probably find a room to rent in a damp and drafty room above the dirt paved-street. With limited resources, he would probably join other immigrants crowded into bunks.

With the Industrial Revolution taking hold, factories were popping up in cities all over the growing nation to support increasing populations domestically and abroad. The immigrant would probably find work in a factory, working in tight quarters with other immigrants in the sweltering heat for twelve to sixteen hours a day. As they would work side by side, the noise of a hacking cough of a man would be inaudible over the rumble of dangerous machines. Barely able to work from fatigue, the immigrant would try to keep pace with another twenty-year-old pushing the odds of his life expectancy next to him. With the likes of tuberculosis now spreading between men, they would probably carry with them this deadly bacterium back to the crowded streets. As the group of immigrants trudged back through the streets filled with decay, they would probably quickly take a scoop of water from a barrel to relieve their cough. However, the water would probably be contaminated by the likes of rats feasting in the dirty streets. All these things would probably cause the immigrant to die early.

You would probably argue that even with Ellis Island around, an immigrant would face the same realities of unsanitary homes, poor working conditions and contaminated food and water. Yes, but with Ellis Island's provision of holistic help – medical, mental, and social – the immigrant would have a higher chance of survival or having a longer life post arrival. In fact, it is not crazy to say that Ellis Island might have contributed to the increasing life expectancy at the turn of the 19th century. Data would show that "until the mid-nineteenth century, life expectancy at birth averaged 20 years worldwide, owing mostly to childhood fevers."[43] However, a shift began in the latter part of the 19th century where "life expectancy started to increase in the early industrialized countries while it stayed low in the rest of the world."[44]

Indeed, without Ellis Island, immigrants

would probably have shorter lives. Worse, they would probably carry with them diseases from their home countries, spreading them amid the already disease-infested New York City. In such a scenario, immigration to America would probably decline, if not altogether halted by the government. With fear of outbreaks, locals on one hand would be wary of more sick immigrants coming in, while immigrants, on the other hand, would be scared of the health disaster awaiting them in America. What a tragic image! Without Ellis Island, the island where it stands today would have remained as Gibbet Island, with a swaying pirate hanging from the gallows warning an immigrant of the challenges and tragedy ahead. The only immigrants this rocky island would have ever seen would be the Canada geese migrating each year.

    Thus, had Ellis Island washed away, America would not have the same level of medical awareness and sophistication in handling infectious diseases. There are indeed parallels to be drawn between Ellis Island's fight against contagious diseases with our very recent combat with the Covid-19 pandemic. In both instances, we see doctors and nurses on the front line, observing safety precautions in the form of, among others, quarantine to slow the spread of the infection. Employing techniques such as sterilization, disinfection and setting up isolation facilities, while instinctive today, were novel innovative methods during the time of Ellis Island. The medical practices at Ellis Island, coupled with the rapid spread of knowledge and information, contributed to our ability today to tackle some of the greatest medical challenges just like the recent deadly pandemic.

Had Ellis Island washed away, America would have also lacked the manpower and talent it needed to build infrastructure spanning coast to coast and to rise as a global superpower. Records note that roughly one in three Americans can trace their history to Ellis Island. Thus, if these immigrants never arrived through this port of entry, the United States population in 1940 could possibility have been 80 million versus the 120 million that the US Census Bureau recorded right before war broke out abroad. And with 1 in 10 members of the population fighting in World War II, that would mean having only 8 million troops versus 12 million. As a large part of the population was already malnourished coming out of the Great Depression, it could be that the United States would have been ill-prepared to send its strong population to fight. Without immigrants to farm or to fight, America would never have been able to rise up to fight off tyranny. I can go one step further. In 1940, Pew Research records that the United States population was 8.5% 1st generation Americans.[45] What if this population never came to America and was abroad fighting on the wrong side? For sure, the world would look very different today if America was not able to build and supply such a military force.

Had Ellis Island washed away, America would not have been a land of cultural diversity. Indeed, the immigrants who passed through Ellis Island carried with them their native languages, cultures, religions and way of life. Immigration then facilitated the free travel of ideas and information, enriching the social and cultural dynamics in America. Even today, as a runner who had the opportunity to run the five boroughs of New York City, I remember that marathoners are encouraged to take in the diverse cultural sites and the smell of different cuisines representing various nations of the world. Unique cultures still abound and are still embraced not only in the big cities but in each small community where families of immigrants settled in.

Had Ellis Island washed away, America would not have been known as the land of opportunity. During the days of Ellis Island, aid societies and religious leaders demonstrated on the shores of the island that America was a place of opportunity and acceptance, a place where immigrants could dream bigger without fear. Of course, the process was not perfect from the get-go. The demands for a literacy test, measuring the circumference of a person's head, and the use of the terms 'idiot' and 'imbecile' show that the process was far from perfect. However, I would like to believe that immigration legislations over the years have improved, and hopefully will continue to improve, as we realize that America was founded on the principle of giving everyone the right to pursue happiness and that all men were created equal. Today, "44.9 million immigrants (foreign-born individuals) comprised 14 percent of the national population" as this is still a nation of immigrants chasing that 'American Dream.'[46]

Thankfully, Ellis Island was not simply washed away. Thankfully, when immigrant families came to America from 1892 to 1954, they found Ellis Island built (or being built) with a growing city to the east and cantilevers stretching out in the distance building homes, factories, and even hospitals. Thankfully, as families waited for their ferry into the city, Red Cross aid workers were there handing small loaves of crusty bread to aid families on the journey. Thankfully, as these families broke bread for the first time in a place they have never been before, they experienced on American soil what was written in Matthew 25:35: "I was hungry and you gave me food, I was thirsty and you gave me drink, I was a stranger and you welcomed me."

It is perhaps in realizing that we are all immigrants in a temporary home that we can welcome and love each other well even today. May we continue the Ellis Island hallmark of welcoming people into our land, stretching out a hand to those who want to pursue a better fulfilled life regardless of where they are from.

AFTERWORD

"For time and the world do not stand still"
– John F. Kennedy

After safely guiding a tour through the Contagious Disease Hospital at Ellis Island, we step out onto the lawn by what would become the Chief of Medicine's House. The beautiful home would be constructed at the southeastern most corner of the island with the very best view of the Statue of Liberty. The last stop being a home and not a hospital room seems like an oddity from my previous medical history facts and attempts at humorous jokes. But the oddity is when the group finally steps outside and is transported back to modern time. The cityscape across the harbor is now the choice for family photos while the sun glints off their polished white hardhats. I often remind my guests to not forget the history that they had not only heard, but seen in the hospitals.

I have had the privilege of exploring more of these buildings than probably most. When I joined Save Ellis Island in 2016, the group of volunteer guides was seldom above a dozen and it was joked, when I joined, that I brought down the group's average age considerably. These amazing volunteers, many of them were former leaders in their industries, were dedicating their time and energy to save buildings that, in many cases, our own families had never even used for their immigration story. Recall that the peak years of Ellis Island ran a short fourteen years in the early 1900's.

However, as time passed, the size of our tour groups grew larger, our volunteer count increased, and we always felt like we stood a real chance of one day reaching the $500 million needed to restore these buildings even if we knew that number was climbing. The figure was often our point of reference to thank our guests for their ticket purchase. In the spring of 2020 though, it all came to a screeching halt as our interest in medical history was truly brought to the present-day concern which was the Covid-19 pandemic. Tours would cease, guides would move, and time would continue to claim these buildings.

Today, tours have resumed, allowing photographers to capture the arrested decay, grandchildren of Ellis Island immigrants to feel closer to their ancestors, and Scout Troops and modern-day doctors to see these remarkable spaces. But with each broken window, freezing and thawing of the concrete, these pieces of history show why it is in fact a 'hard-hat' tour if only for a precaution. Today, efforts continue to make these tours fully open, with repairs, and guides always being on the watch, but time will certainly not stand still.

This summer, this upcoming holiday long-weekend, put on your hiking boots and go explore. In 2016, the National Parks Service celebrated their 100th anniversary serving our nation. They encouraged people to 'go find your park.' I encourage you to do the same. With 423 National Parks protecting over 84 million acres of wild landscapes and historic sites, there is certainly an option for anybody. And if you are fortunate enough to go to Ellis Island and meet Park Ranger Sam, introduce your children to these servant leaders in the parks and protect these spaces for future generations.

But even if you don't get the amazing chance to go take a tour of the hospitals at Ellis Island, at least take a look across the ferry slip as you board your ferry home. As the sun sets behind the hospital buildings, the sunshine beautifully reflects off the Spanish terracotta roofs and leaves long shadows from the deep-rooted American sycamore trees wrapped around the buildings. Ellis Island was the beginning of so many American stories and the histories that this place allowed to happen shall never be forgotten.

ACKNOWLEDGEMENT

It is my utmost pleasure to stand on the shoulders of giants who have had a love for immigration history. I wish to thank beyond measure the authors cited in the source notes. Over the years, I have been so fortunate to have the support of good friends at Save Ellis Island such as Pat Montlary, John McInnes, and the late John Malczynski who mentored me in the halls of the hospitals. But I am most indebted to Jim Peskin who truly leads all the guides with such vigor and passion as well as Tori Brouhard for her dedicated fact finding. My work alongside such an inspiring group of docents has been such a gift. The work to not only restore the hospitals, but to tell the stories of those who came before us is never in vain.

I also would like to acknowledge the wonderful mentors and leaders of the National Parks Service. Without the privilege given by the National Parks Service for us to lead tours to the south side of Ellis Island, I would be at a loss. I could never thank enough Michael Amato, Peter Wong, and my favorite and dear friend, Sam Webb, for their leadership and friendship at Ellis Island. Their dedication to preserving Ellis Island, the Statue of Liberty and all our national treasures is valued beyond measure. Also, a humble thanks to Charlie DeLeo, the Keeper of the Flame, for our times in prayer and exploration of the Island together.

To Shane and Alana Kiefer, thank you for the beautiful photography that will provide readers of this book a view of the Ellis Island today. Your eye for the beauty in this world is beyond compare.

To my family, thank you for always encouraging my love of history and allowing me to be a Renaissance man.

I also extend my thanks to the Hoboken Grace Dinner group that encouraged me to write on and to the whole Hoboken Grace Church family for their support and prayers in my endeavors.

And lastly, to my Grace. Thank you for always encouraging, inspiring me, believing in me, laughing through our editing, and supporting me. My deepest and greatest appreciation is forever yours.

BIBLIOGRAPHY

1) https://poets.org/poem/new-colossus?gclid=Cj0KCQiAubmPBhCyARIsAJWNpiNwpDRBM1h62M4hLcNJlgiPrQHBuVd6g1RG9_H_TwJAxsmcrbNtJakaAjoeEALw_wcB
2) https://www.gjenvick.com/FAQs/HowFastCouldASteamshipCrossTheOcean.html#:~:text=Their%20efficiency%20may%20be%20said,6%20days%20and%2020%20minutes.
3) https://catalogs.marinersmuseum.org/object/CL4604
4) https://www.smithsonianmag.com/history/true-native-new-yorkers-can-never-truly-reclaim-their-homeland-180970472/
5) https://www.nypl.org/blog/2011/06/01/history-half-shell-intertwined-story-new-york-city-and-its-oysters
6) https://daily.jstor.org/the-curious-history-of-ellis-island/
7) https://www.history.com/news/9-things-you-may-not-know-about-ellis-island
8) https://www.nps.gov/elis/learn/historyculture/ellis-island-chronology.htm
9) https://migrationmemorials.trinity.duke.edu/items/fort-gibson-other-ellis-island-story

10) https://www.fbi.gov/history/famous-cases/black-tom-1916-bombing
11) https://www.encyclopedia.com/history/encyclopedias-almanacs-transcripts-and-maps/populations-great-britain-and-america
12) https://www.census.gov/programs-surveys/geography/guidance/geo-areas/urban-rural/ua-facts.html
13) https://ourworldindata.org/urbanization#long-run-history-of-urbanization
14) https://www.worldatlas.com/articles/how-many-shipwrecks-are-there.html
15) https://www.post-gazette.com/local/pittsburgh-history/2014/03/02/Eyewitness-1855-Rail-and-factory-workers-died-on-average-at-age-27/stories/201403020066
16) https://www.nps.gov/cacl/learn/historyculture/index.htm
17) https://www.census.gov/programs-surveys/decennial-census/decade.1820.html
18) https://www.history.com/news/steerage-act-immigration-19th-century
19) Porter. Greatest Benefit to Mankind. WW Norton, 1999.
20) https://www.uscis.gov/about-us/our-history/overview-of-ins-history/early-american-immigration-policies
21) https://southstreetseaportmuseum.org/castle-clinton/
22) Kapp, Friedrich. Immigration, and the Commissioners of Emigration of the State of New York. Gale, Sabin Americana, 2012.
23) http://npshistory.com/publications/stli/clr-

ellis-island.pdf
24) https://www.history.com/news/remembering-annie-moore-ellis-islands-first-immigrant
25) https://www.nytimes.com/2006/09/14/nyregion/14annie.html
26) https://www.archives.gov/education/lessons/immigration.html
27) https://www.marinehospital.org/publichealth.htm
28) Rutkow, Ira M. Seeking the Cure: A History of Medicine in America. Scribner, 2012.
29) Conway, Lorie. Forgotten Ellis Island: The Extraordinary Story of America's Immigrant Hospital. 1st ed., Smithsonian, 2007.
30) https://millercenter.org/the-presidency/presidential-speeches/december-3-1901-first-annual-message
31) https://www.cdc.gov/healthywater/drinking/history.html
32) https://journalofethics.ama-assn.org/article/medical-examination-immigrants-ellis-island/2008-04
33) The Modern Hospital. July 1917 ed., IX, McGraw-Hill.
34) https://www.cdc.gov/tb/worldtbday/history.htm
35) https://nursing-theory.org/nursing-theorists/Florence-Nightingale.php
36) https://immigrationhistory.org/item/1917-barred-zone-act/
37) http://npshistory.com/publications/stli/clr-ellis-island.pdf
38) http://digitalexhibits.wsulibs.wsu.edu/exhibits/show/immigration-impacts-in-the-pac/immigration-west-movement-labor

39) https://www.history.com/news/last-hired-first-fired-how-the-great-depression-affected-african-americans
40) https://www.nps.gov/elis/learn/historyculture/people_immigrant_aid_worker.htm
41) https://www.nytimes.com/2010/04/29/nyregion/29lost.html
42) Bellevue Hospital, Edwin M. Knights Jr., M.D., History Magazine http://www.history-magazine.com/bellevue.html
43) https://www.ncbi.nlm.nih.gov/pmc/articles/PMC4980761/
44) https://ourworldindata.org/life-expectancy
45) https://www.pewresearch.org/hispanic/chart/first-and-second-generation-share-of-the-population/
46) https://www.americanimmigrationcouncil.org/research/immigrants-in-the-united-states

ABOUT THE AUTHOR

Brett Moyer

Brett Moyer has been an avid docent, as well as a medical historian tour guide, in the Ellis Island Immigrant Hospitals since 2016. He is also a member of the Warrior Run Fort Freeland Heritage Society since 2001 where 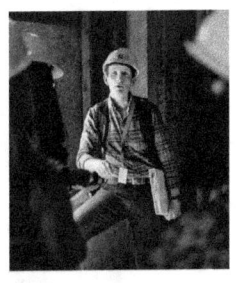 he serves as a master craftsman rake maker. He is a 2013 graduate of Susquehanna University and has worked in corporate finance for the nation's biggest banks since then. He continues to pursue his passion for history and giving back to his local community. In 2021, he released his first book, Had Lincoln Lived, which has been internationally recognized.

amazon.com/author/brettmoyer

www.ingramcontent.com/pod-product-compliance
Lightning Source LLC
Chambersburg PA
CBHW071510220526
45472CB00003B/967